Field Guide to
Clinical
Dermatology

2nd Edition

DAVID H. FRANKEL, M.D.

Assistant Clinical Professor of Dermatology
Mount Sinai School of Medicine

Assistant Attending,
New York Methodist Hospital

Dermatologist,
UNITE HERE Health Center

Medical Editor,
The Journal of Urban Health
New York Academy of Medicine
New York, New York

Lippincott Williams & Wilkins
a Wolters Kluwer business
Philadelphia · Baltimore · New York · London
Buenos Aires · Hong Kong · Sydney · Tokyo

Acquisitions Editor: Sonya Seigafuse
Managing Editor: Nancy Winter
Project Manager: Jennifer Harper
Manufacturing Coordinator: Kathleen Brown
Marketing Director: Sharon Zinner
Design Coordinator: Stephen Druding
Cover Designer: Larry Didona
Production Services: Laserwords Private Limited
Printer: R.R. Donnelley, Shenzhen China

Library of Congress Cataloging-in-Publication Data

Field guide to clinical dermatology / [edited by] David H. Frankel.—2nd ed.
    p. ; cm.
    Includes index.
    ISBN 0-7817-5627-8
    1. Skin—Diseases—Handbooks, manuals, etc. 2. Primary care (Medicine)—Handbooks,
manuals, etc. I. Frankel, David H. II. Title. [DNLM: 1. Skin Diseases—diagnosis—Handbooks.
2. Skin Diseases—therapy—Handbooks. WR 39 F454 2007]

RL74.F54 2007
616.5—dc22

                                                                            2006008353

    Care has been taken to confirm the accuracy of the information presented
and to describe generally accepted practices. However, the authors, editors, and
publisher are not responsible for errors or omissions or for any consequences
from application of the information in this book and make no warranty, expressed
or implied, with respect to the currency, completeness, or accuracy of the contents
of the publication. Application of this information in a particular situation
remains the professional responsibility of the practitioner.
    The authors, editors, and publisher have exerted every effort to ensure that
drug selection and dosage set forth in this text are in accordance with current
recommendations and practice at the time of publication. However, in view of
ongoing research, changes in government regulations, and the constant flow of
information relating to drug therapy and drug reactions, the reader is urged to
check the package insert for each drug for any change in indications and dosage
and for added warnings and precautions. This is particularly important when the
recommended agent is a new or infrequently employed drug.
    Some drugs and medical devices presented in this publication have Food and
Drug Administration (FDA) clearance for limited use in restricted research
settings. It is the responsibility of the health care provider to ascertain the FDA
status of each drug or device planned for use in their clinical practice.
    To purchase additional copies of this book, call our customer service
department at (800) 638-3030 or fax orders to (301) 223-2320. International
customers should call (301) 223-2300.
    Visit Lippincott Williams & Wilkins on the Internet: at LWW.com. Lippincott
Williams & Wilkins customer service representatives are available from 8:30 am to
6 pm, EST.

                                            10 9 8 7 6 5 4 3 2 1

This edition is given for love of Julia and Eli,
my children.
It is for my mother, my brothers and for Annie.
And it is from my heart to the memory of
Robert Frankel, M.D.,
my father.

CONTENTS

B. *Red rashes on the face*

C. *Red rashes (not face)*

D. *Scaling rashes*

SECTION III ■ BLISTERS

SECTION IV ■ BUMPS

A. Bumps you think may be cancer

E. Red bumps that hurt

F. Scars

G. Soft, mushy bumps or lumps

H. Yellow bumps

SECTION V ▪ SPOTS

A. Purple (it won't blanch)

GUIDE TO THE BOOK

CONTRIBUTING AUTHORS

Jeffrey P. Callen, M.D. *Professor, Department of Medicine (Dermatology); Chief, Division of Dermatology, University of Louisville, Louisville, Kentucky*

John T. Crissey, M.D. *Clinical Professor, Department of Medicine (Dermatology), University of Southern California School of Medicine; Attending Dermatologist, Department of Medicine (Dermatology), University of Southern California Medical Center, Los Angeles, California*

David H. Frankel, M.D. *Assistant Clinical Professor, Department of Dermatology, Mount Sinai School of Medicine; Assistant Attending, New York Methodist Hospital; Dermatologist, UNITE HERE Health Center; Medical Editor, The Journal of Urban Health, New York Academy of Medicine, New York, New York*

Charles A. Gropper, M.D. *Associate Clinical Professor, Department of Dermatology, Mount Sinai School of Medicine, New York; Chief, Department of Dermatology, Bronx Veterans Affairs Medical Center and St. Barnabas Hospital, Bronx, New York*

David J. Leffell, M.D. *Professor, Chief, Section of Dermatologic Surgery and Cutaneous Oncology, Department of Dermatology and Surgery, Yale School of Medicine, New Haven, Connecticut*

Larry E. Millikan, M.D., F.A.C.P. *Professor, Chair Emeritus, Department of Dermatology, Tulane University School of Medicine, New Orleans, Louisiana*

Lawrence Charles Parish, M.D. *Clinical Professor, Department of Dermatology and Cutaneous Biology, Director, Jefferson Center for International Dermatology, Jefferson Medical College of Thomas Jefferson University; Chief, Department of Dermatology, The Frankford Hospitals, Philadelphia, Pennsylvania; Visiting Professor, Department of Dermatology, Tulane University School of Medicine, New Orleans, Louisiana*

Andrew J. Scheman, M.D. *Associate Professor, Department of Clinical Dermatology, Northwestern University Medical Center, Chicago, Illinois*

James C. Shaw, M.D., F.R.C.P.C. *Associate Professor, Division of Dermatology, University of Toronto, Toronto Western Hospital, University Health Network, Toronto, Ontario, Canada*

PREFACE TO THE FIRST EDITION

This book is for primary-care practitioners. It is meant as a working manual, to be carried and used daily. It is deliberately long on direct, clinical content and short on pathogenesis and etiology. I hope it helps.

The medication dosages given in this book are for adult patients, unless otherwise noted. The dosages must therefore be adjusted for pediatric patients.

The Table of Contents and the Guide to the Book organize the text. I know it is a bit unorthodox. However, as an internist and dermatologist who has always practiced among primary-care professionals, I find that the standard dermatology algorithms are often a bit too long and confusing to be easily learned. I have therefore tried to organize the contents to reflect the predominance of two simple categories: what the patient says (e.g., "it itches"), or what you see (e.g., a red rash).

Of course, itch is subjective, red rashes scale, scaling rashes are red, and no algorithm is perfect. Therefore, only the predominant symptom or sign is the one that gets the title in the Guide to the Book. Please read the entire Guide to the Book. Most of the skin diseases you will see are listed there.

David H. Frankel, M.D.
Brooklyn, New York
October, 1998

PREFACE TO THE SECOND EDITION

"Five years have past; five summers, with the length/Of five long winters!"[1] Well—seven, actually—have come and gone since the Preface to the first edition. In those years I married, began a family with twins, and moved from full-time medical journalism and editorship and started a full time private practice in dermatology. Should there be any further commotion in my life over the next seven years I'm sure I'll have no energy left for a third edition!

I am grateful for the success of the book. Doctors in the United States and abroad have responded well to both its style and instruction and so we present a second edition. To be sure, there have been significant changes in dermatology over the interval. Nonetheless, the basics of caring for patients with skin diseases remain the same in many ways. My goal in this edition has been to meld the changes to the basics. As I said before, I hope it helps.

I have dedicated this book to my father, as best I can. I regret I lack the perfect words to capture our loss at his passing this March, and I wish Julia and Eli had the years to know him better. Long ago, my father and mother saw my early interest in poetry and made a present of a volume I keep. And from that, once again, Wordsworth has the better sense of it all: "To me the meanest flower that blows can give/Thoughts that do often lie too deep for tears."[2]

David H. Frankel, M.D.
Brooklyn, New York
October, 2005

[1] Lines composed a few miles above Tintern Abbey, on revisiting the banks of the Wye during a tour, July 13, 1798; William Wordsworth. The English romantic poets. Marius Bewley, ed. Modern Library Books. New York, 1970, p 149.

[2] "Ode; intimations of immortality from recollections of early childhood," William Wordsworth; ibid, p 198.

ACKNOWLEDGMENTS

Once again I thank the contributing authors of this book. They continue to share their enthusiasm for the unusual approach we have taken and have given themselves generously till its completion. I could do no better in my career than to have friends and colleagues of their grace and ability. Nancy Winter of Lippincott Williams & Wilkins is an editor of skill—and unending patience. Dr. David Vlahov of the New York Academy of Medicine has been a true friend and colleague. Drs. Alan Lorincz and Maria Medenica are the heroes of any clinical successes I may have with my patients. I feel their kind and patient instruction each day I step into practice. Dr. Robin Fox, my former editor at *The Lancet*, gave me opportunities that I will never forget and can never repay. I am fortunate, always, to have Joel Bennett as my friend.

Section I

Warning: A Note on Topical Steroids

Chapter 1

PROPER USE OF TOPICAL CORTICOSTEROIDS

Andrew J. Scheman

WARNING

It is unusual to begin a pharmacology or formulary section with a warning. Warnings are generally reserved for the end. But because topical corticosteroids often cause serious local side effects when used improperly and because prescriptions are sometimes given in a cavalier manner, it is worth describing pitfalls at the outset.

Local side effects of steroid use can be permanent, disfiguring, and very distressing. Skin atrophied from topical corticosteroids appears thin, transparent, shiny, hypopigmented, and telangiectatic (Fig. 1–1). Striae may develop. These changes are especially noticeable and distressing on the face. Other high-risk areas prone to steroid atrophy are intertriginous areas, such as the groin, axillae, neck, and intergluteal cleft.

It is worth remembering that topical corticosteroids may cause the same systemic side effects as oral corticosteroids. This is especially true in children, in whom the high ratio of skin surface area to body weight makes treatment of even relatively small areas of the skin more problematic.

Figure 1–1 Atrophy from topical corticosteroids presents as thin, hypopigmented, telangiectatic skin.

Patients—or their family members—often use whatever cream is in the medicine cabinet. It is not unusual for a patient with acne to use a super-potent topical corticosteroid on the cheek or nose, believing that "one cream is just as good as another." Therefore, it is wise to prescribe only the amount that the patient needs immediately and to limit refills.

Although it sounds simplistic, patients on potent topical medications need follow-up no less than patients taking oral medications. Proper and timely adjustments of therapy to less (or more) potent preparations hastens relief from skin disease and limits the potential for untoward effects.

AVOIDING TOPICAL CORTICOSTEROID SIDE EFFECTS IN HIGH-RISK AREAS

Unfortunately, we all encounter instances in which a dermatitis on the face, groin, axillae, or intergluteal folds, or on a child, does not respond to lowest-potent agents. As will be discussed, low- or medium-potent topical corticosteroids that are nonfluorinated can be effective in this situation; desonide 0.05%, and, if a more potent agent is needed, hydrocortisone valerate 0.2%, are good choices. Occasionally, an even stronger preparation is needed. Mometasone furoate 0.1% ointment is the only high-potent topical corticosteroid ointment that is nonfluorinated. Caution is still in order, however. Although the use of nonfluorinated topical corticosteroids reduces the likelihood of side effects, it does not eliminate them.

TOPICAL CORTICOSTEROIDS ARE GROUPED BY STRENGTH

The list of topical corticosteroids has many chemical names that may be unfamiliar to you, and prednisone—probably the most commonly used systemic corticosteroid—is missing. This is because prednisone, like most systemic corticosteroids, is weak as an ointment or cream. When a fluorinated side chain is added to the basic steroid molecule, these glucocorticoids are more effective as topical agents. Unfortunately, the fluorinated side chains also increase the potential for side effects. Indeed, many of today's topical corticosteroids can be dangerous when they are used incorrectly.

The strength of a topical corticosteroid is measured by its ability to produce vasoconstriction—the Stoughton assay. The more vasoconstriction that occurs, the more potent the steroid is. On the basis of the vasoconstriction model, topical corticosteroids are divided into seven categories. Class 1 is the strongest, and class 7 is the weakest. For the purposes of this book, we label only five groups: (a) "super-potent," (b) "high-potent," (c) "medium-potent," (d) "low-potent," and (e) "lowest-potent/over-the-counter."

The strength of a topical corticosteroid is related to the potency of the steroid molecule. However, it is also related to the base, or vehicle, in which it is compounded. Ointments are often stronger than creams. Generic products may be a bit weaker than their branded "equivalents," but they are often considerably cheaper.

WHAT THE POTENCY GROUPS MEAN IN PRACTICE

Super-potent topical corticosteroids must be used with great caution. These fluorinated agents should be used only for limited eruptions (less than 10% of the body) on non–high-risk areas. They should not be used for more than 2 to 3 weeks and not in children at all. After the acute eruption has been brought under control, it is wise to switch to a lower-strength preparation for maintenance therapy.

High-potent topical corticosteroids are usually fluorinated. Their use should be limited to small eruptions, and they should not be used on high-risk areas or on children. However, high-potent preparations can be used for longer periods than the super-potent products and are indicated for maintenance therapy in severe, localized inflammatory skin problems. Again, their use must be closely supervised.

Medium-potent, **fluorinated** topical corticosteroids are used to control severe, widespread inflammatory dermatoses or to treat less severe, localized conditions. Medium-potent, **nonfluorinated** agents can be used for severe dermatoses of the face, groin, axilla, and intergluteal cleft, and on children.

Low-potent, **fluorinated** topical corticosteroids are used for moderately severe, inflammatory widespread dermatoses. Low-potent **nonfluorinated** agents are safer on the high-risk areas and on children.

Lowest-potent and over-the-counter preparations can be used on the high-risk areas and on children. Although hydrocortisone 2.5% would seem to be much stronger than hydrocortisone 1%, it is only marginally so. The 2.5% preparation is available by prescription only. Hydrocortisone 1% is the weakest topical corticosteroid that seems to be clinically effective; hydrocortisone 0.5% is of little benefit. Both are available over the counter.

A note of warning: some compounded products can surprise you. Lotrisone cream, one of the most widely prescribed topical medications for fungal infections, contains betamethasone dipropionate 0.05% in addition to the antifungal agent clotrimazole. Another "antifungal," Mycolog II, contains triamcinolone acetonide 0.1% in addition to the antifungal agent nystatin. Although these agents are often regarded as antifungals alone, they should not be used on high-risk areas or on children because they contain strong and potentially harmful fluorinated corticosteroids.

CHOOSING THE VEHICLE: OINTMENT, CREAM, OR SOLUTION?

An *ointment* is a heavy, occlusive, non–water-containing vehicle, which provides significant moisturization. **Creams** are emulsions of oil and water that are less moisturizing and dissolve more rapidly into the skin than ointments. Creams that are predominantly oil-based provide more moisturization than those that are predominantly water-based; oil-free creams are the least moisturizing. **Solutions** are liquid forms of topical corticosteroid in which the liquid vehicle is usually alcohol, water, or propylene glycol.

For dry-skin conditions such as chronic atopic dermatitis, an ointment is best. For inflammatory dermatoses in which dry skin does not play a major role, such as contact dermatitis, creams are best. For oily dermatoses such as seborrheic dermatitis or for inflammatory conditions in areas of thick hair growth, solutions are best. Solutions can also be used on the face underneath cosmetics. Although some solutions are classified as super-, high-, or medium-potent solutions, they are relatively safe for long-term use on the scalp. However, it is wise to examine the scalp periodically to make sure that atrophy does not develop.

APPLICATION SCHEDULE AND AMOUNT TO DISPENSE

Topical corticosteroids are used twice daily. The amount dispensed varies by body habitus, but a rough measure for dispensing is shown in Table 1–1. See Appendix A for a list of topical agents and their brand names.

TABLE 1-1 Guidelines for Dispensing Topical Corticosteroids

Location	Amount Dispensed (2 × daily for 1 week) (g)[a]
Face or neck	15
Chest or back	45
Hands (both)	15
Arm (one)	30
Feet (both)	30
Leg (one)	60
Entire body	180–240

[a] For children, reduce the amount dispensed proportional to adult body size.

Appendix A

Topical Corticosteroid Agents

Strength	Brand
Ointments	
Super-potent	
Augmented betamethasone dipropionate 0.05%	Diprolene
Clobetasol propionate 0.05%	Temovate
Diflorasone diacetate 0.05%	Psorcon
Halobetasol propionate 0.05%	Ultravate
High-potent	
Fluocinonide 0.05%	Lidex
Mometasone furoate 0.1%[a]	Elocon
Desoximetasone 0.25%	Topicort
Betamethasone dipropionate 0.05%	Diprosone
Medium-potent	
Betamethasone valerate 0.1%	Beta-val
Hydrocortisone valerate 0.2%[a]	Westcort
Triamcinolone acetonide 0.1%	Aristocort
Low-potent	
Desonide 0.05%[a]	DesOwen, Tridesilon
Triamcinolone acetonide 0.025%	Aristocort, Kenalog
Lowest-potent/over-the-counter	
Hydrocortisone 2.5%[a]	Hytone
Hydrocortisone 1.0%[a]	Over-the-counter
Creams	
Super-potent	
Clobetasol propionate 0.055%	Temovate
Halobetasol propionate 0.05%	Ultravate
High-potent	
Augmented betamethasone dipropionate 0.05%	Diprolene
Desoximetasone 0.25%	Topicort
Diflorasone diacetate 0.05%	Florone, Psorcon
Fluocinonide 0.05%	Lidex

Appendix A *(Continued)*

Medium-potent	
Mometasone furoate 0.1%[a]	Elocon
Hydrocortisone valerate 0.2%[a]	Westcort
Triamcinolone acetonide 0.1%	Aristocort, Kenalog
Low-potent	
Desonide 0.05%[a]	DesOwen, Tridesilon
Fluocinolone acetonide 0.01%	Synalar
Lowest-potent/over-the-counter	
Hydrocortisone 2.5%[a]	Hytone
Hydrocortisone 1.0%[a]	Over-the-counter

Solutions

Super-potent	
Clobetasol propionate 0.05%	Temovate
High-potent	
Fluocinonide 0.05%	Lidex
Medium-potent	
Betamethasone valerate 0.01%	Betatrex
Betamethasone dipropionate 0.05%	Diprosone
Low-potent	
Fluocinolone acetonide 0.025%	Synalar
Lowest-potent/over-the-counter	
Hydrocortisone 1.0%[a]	Over-the-counter

Dozens of prescription topical corticosteroids are on the market, and new ones keep emerging. As a rule, generic preparations are far less expensive than branded products. Therefore, many of the products listed are generic preparations, although brand names are given for the sake of convenience.

[a] Nonfluorinated.

Rashes

Chapter 2

ATOPIC DERMATITIS
(ICD-9 691.8)

Lawrence Charles Parish

SYMPTOMS AND SIGNS

The hallmark of atopic dermatitis (AD) is itching, which can be severe. AD is characterized by redness, scaling, and lichenification. In adults, it most commonly occurs in the antecubital and popliteal fossae (Figs. 2–1 and 2–2) and on the nape of the neck. Because there is no true primary lesion, patients with AD often present solely with itching or so-called sensitive skin. As the skin is scratched or rubbed to obtain relief, it may show excoriations, vesiculation, and crusting. Secondary bacterial infection of the skin is common.

Presentation of AD is variable, depending on the age of the patient. In infants and children, the redness and scaling may be on the extensor surfaces, face, or trunk. Infantile AD may be short-lived or may be a prodrome to lifelong dermatitis. As the child grows older, the traditional flexor areas become involved.

Patients with AD often have hyperlinear palms (Fig. 2–3) and infraorbital creases, so-called Dennie–Morgan folds. Rubbing of the lips creates cracking and surrounding erythema, known as the **furrowed mouth syndrome**. In older

Figure 2–1 Atopic dermatitis. Antecubital erythema and lichenification are hallmarks of the disease.

Figure 2–2   Atopic dermatitis. Typical appearance in the popliteal fossae with postinflammatory hyperpigmentation.

Figure 2–3   Hyperlinear palms are a clue to the diagnosis of atopic dermatitis.

Figure 2-4 Keratosis pilaris. Hyperkeratotic follicular papules on the extensor upper aspect of the arms feel like sandpaper and respond to lactic acid cream or lotion.

patients or during times of quiescence, the only manifestations of AD may be dryness and scaling—erythema crackle.

Associated conditions include pityriasis alba, in which there are irregular patches of scaling and hypopigmentation, and **keratosis pilaris (KP)**, the almost physiologic hyperkeratotic accentuation of hair follicles on the lateral and posterior upper arms and on the anterior thighs (Fig. 2–4). KP presents as firm red or skin-colored papules, giving a "sandpaper" feel to the area. African-American patients may also have perifollicular accentuation like goose flesh.

DIFFERENTIAL DIAGNOSIS

Seborrheic dermatitis is usually limited to the scalp, glabella, and perinasal area. Contact dermatitis, especially when it is on the hands, can mimic AD. The history helps in achieving a diagnosis. Neurodermatitis has a similar morphology and sometimes more varied distribution, but the distinguishing feature is the lack of atopic history—asthma, allergic rhinitis, or eczema in the patient or in a relative. Redness and scaling on the feet may suggest tinea pedis; however, children rarely have a dermatophyte infection, and the lack of interdigital involvement rules out a fungal infection.

HOW TO MAKE THE DIAGNOSIS

Although AD may result in eosinophilia or elevated immunoglobulin E (IgE) levels, the diagnosis is made by observation and the personal or family history of atopy. Hyperlinear palms and Dennie–Morgan fold are helpful clues. White dermatographism, in which stroking the skin gives a raised white line, is common.

TREATMENT

The most important aspect of therapy is to "put the skin to rest" by avoiding irritants. Soap should be limited to the critical areas—hands, face, axillae, and groin. Excessively hot water is also destructive to the skin. Patients will want to bathe daily, but extensive soaking may aggravate their skin. Short, lukewarm showers are acceptable.

Topical corticosteroids are needed for long periods. Therefore, high-potent and super-potent ointments or creams should be limited to flares, and medium-potent or low-potent agents should be used for maintenance. Topical immunomodulators can be helpful in the treatment of AD but should be used with caution because of the current U.S. Food and Drug Administration (FDA) "black-box" warning on increased risk of neoplasia associated with the use of these agents. Oral corticosteroids should be reserved for severe flares. Prednisone, 30 mg daily for 10 days, may break the cycle. Colloidal baths initially reduce itching, whereas oral antihistamines relieve pruritus but do not affect the natural course of this chronic dermatitis.

Patients should be encouraged to use unscented moisturizers. Creams or ointments are more effective than lotions and should be applied immediately after showering to limit irritation and drying, which inevitably results from soap and water. This is especially important in winter. Remember that the sensitivity of patients with AD to wool carries over into lanolin-based products. Lipid-free products are safest. In hot, humid weather, secondary bacterial infection may require a course of antistaphylococcal oral antimicrobial agents such as erythromycin, 250 mg three times daily for 7 to 10 days.

KP responds to lactic acid 12% cream or lotion or to urea preparations; both are applied twice daily.

PROGNOSIS

There is no way to know how long AD will last. Often, infants and children have AD that never returns in later years. Other patients develop AD in middle age; still others have severe AD for most of their lives. Sometimes, AD surfaces only for certain periods during adulthood. If patients attend to proper skin care, they are less likely to have severe disease if—or when—the condition recurs.

Chapter 3

CONTACT DERMATITIS
(ICD-9 692.9)

Lawrence Charles Parish

SYMPTOMS AND SIGNS

Contact dermatitis causes itching and burning. It is characterized by redness, which can progress to vesiculation, oozing, weeping, scaling, and fissuring. After several days of itching and rubbing, the patient may develop secondary bacterial infection with purulence and crusting in the area. Sometimes, the reaction is so intense that swelling occurs at the contact site and dermatitis occurs at distant sites. The latter phenomenon is called an **id reaction**. Contact dermatitis may be divided into two groups: irritant and allergic.

Irritant contact dermatitis occurs every time the patient comes into contact with the substance. This dermatitis can develop in a few minutes or in several hours. Any person is subject to irritant dermatitis if he or she is in contact with an irritating substance long enough to produce a reaction. The duration of exposure required to produce dermatitis varies. Perhaps the most common contact irritant is soap, especially in the wintertime, when the skin is already dry and irritated. Other common irritants include detergents, cutting oils, solvents, and cement.

Allergic contact dermatitis develops within 24 to 48 hours of exposure to an allergen to which the patient has previously been sensitized. Rhus dermatitis, caused by poison oak, poison ivy, or poison sumac, is the prototypical allergic response. This dermatitis lasts for 10 to 20 days because the rhus oil becomes embedded in the skin. A clue to the diagnosis is its linear pattern. Other common contact allergens include nickel, neomycin, rubber (latex), paraphenylenediamine, lanolin, topical anesthetics, topical antihistamines, and fragrances. It is worth remembering that most metal jewelry contains nickel, even when it is advertised as "solid gold." The alloy is used to strengthen the gold or silver and also to save expenses. Generally, 18-kt gold has an insufficient amount of nickel to cause trouble (Fig. 3–1). Topical neomycin is the most common cause of iatrogenic allergic contact dermatitis.

DIFFERENTIAL DIAGNOSIS

Contact dermatitis is often distinctive because of its localization. Occasionally, it may be confused with atopic dermatitis limited to the antecubital or popliteal fossae or with nummular dermatitis scattered on the body. Because dermatitis on the hands may be nondescript, the term **hand dermatitis** is used to cover a number of dermatitides: atopic, contact, and psoriatic.

HOW TO MAKE THE DIAGNOSIS

The history is most important. If the patient recognizes these symptoms and signs every time he or she has contact with a particular item, then the etiologic battle is won. Sometimes, the offending agent is more difficult to locate, and patch testing is necessary. This involves placing a series of chemicals on the skin, usually the back; covering the applications with a type of nonirritating and nonallergenic dressing such as paper tape; and keeping the area covered for 2 to 3 days. Reaction at the site of the chemical helps confirm the diagnosis.

Figure 3-1 Nickel-causing allergic contact dermatitis from rivet in blue jeans.

TREATMENT

Eliminating the contactant is crucial, although topical corticosteroid ointments and creams are most helpful in reducing the dermatitis. The strength
of the steroid depends on the severity of the dermatitis. With a severe reaction,
such as a reaction to paraphenylenediamine in hair dye or to poison ivy, oral
prednisone, 40 to 60 mg per day for 10 days, may be needed in addition to
high-potent or super-potent topical corticosteroids.

PROGNOSIS

The dermatitis usually clears within a few days after the elimination of the
contactant. Reexposure, particularly chronic reexposure, leads to chronic
dermatitis and lichenification.

Chapter 4

SCABIES
(ICD-9 133.0)

Lawrence Charles Parish

SYMPTOMS AND SIGNS

Scabies causes severe itching, especially at night, when there are fewer distractions. (It is sometimes called the "7-year itch" because it probably lasts 7 years without treatment.) The eruption is characterized by small, 2- to 5-mm red papules that are predominantly found in intertriginous or warm and protected areas such as the finger webs (Fig. 4–1), inframammary areas, and axillae. It is caused by the mite, *Sarcoptes scabiei*. The pathognomonic lesion is the burrow, a brownish, irregular line with scaling at one end and sometimes a vesicle at the other end. Unfortunately, the burrow is often hard to find. Another common site is the penis. Lesions can also appear on the trunk and extremities, but rarely on the face except in children or in immunocompromised patients. The papules sometimes are eczematized and secondarily infected as the result of scratching to alleviate the marked nocturnal itching.

Figure 4–1 Scabies causing burrows in web spaces of the hand.

Figure 4–2 Crusted scabies in a patient with acquired immunodeficiency syndrome (AIDS).

The presentation of scabies can vary. Infants and the elderly can have red papules scattered over the entire body. Crusted scabies represents a severe infestation that occurs in immunocompromised patients (Fig. 4–2). "*Scabies incognito*" occurs when the patient has been applying topical corticosteroids, which impede the inflammatory process but still allow the mites to proliferate.

DIFFERENTIAL DIAGNOSIS

Scabies can be confused with folliculitis and neurodermatitis. Other arthropod bites can look like scabies, but penile lesions confirm the presence of scabies. Canine scabies produces clusters of red papules, usually on the abdomen, but no mites are found on the human skin. Crusted scabies can be confused with eczematous conditions or psoriasis.

HOW TO MAKE THE DIAGNOSIS

A recent lesion is scraped, the material is treated with 10% potassium hydroxide solution to dissolve the keratin, and the specimen is studied under light microscopy. The mite measures 0.4×0.3 mm in females and 0.2×0.15 mm in males (Fig. 4–3). Confirmation may be difficult to obtain if the patient has washed conscientiously with soap.

TREATMENT

Permethrin cream 5% is applied from the neck to the toes for 12 hours before washing it off. A second choice is lindane lotion 1%, applied from the neck to the toes for a 12-hour period before washing it off. Lindane should not be used in infants or in pregnant women. Ivermectin, 200 µg/kg given once, is used as an oral treatment in some countries. To prevent undertreatment or recurrence, topical treatments must be applied to all areas including in the umbilicus and under the fingernails. Symptomatic relief is given with

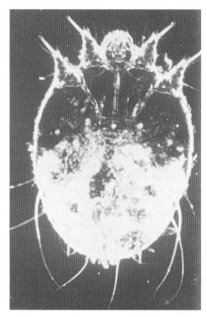

Figure 4–3 *Sarcoptes scaibei* seen under the microscope.

high-potent to super-potent topical corticosteroid ointment or cream. Pruritus can persist even weeks beyond successful therapy.

Treatment should be given to close contacts and family members.

PROGNOSIS

When the application of cream or lotion is inadequate, the condition persists.

Chapter 5

PEDICULOSIS
(ICD-9 132.0 CAPITIS; 132.2 PUBIS; 132.1 CORPORIS)

Lawrence Charles Parish

SYMPTOMS AND SIGNS

Pediculosis can be very pruritic. There are three forms in humans: pediculosis pubis caused by *Phthirus pubis*, pediculosis capitis caused by *Pediculus capitis*, and pediculosis corporis caused by *Pediculus corporis*.

Pediculosis capitis is found only in preadolescent children and almost never in African-American children, for unknown reasons. Scratching can cause a secondary bacterial infection. Crusting appears on the scalp, and excoriations appear on the neck and ears. Occipital and cervical lymph nodes are palpable. Live nits are whitish and shiny and found within 1 cm of the scalp (Fig. 5–1). Dead nits are dull and gray.

Pediculosis pubis is caused by a crab-like organism; hence, the term "crab lice" infestation. The louse grasps the hair and bites the skin, often producing bluish macules 0.5 to 2.5 cm in diameter (maculae cerulea). The nit is 3 to 4 mm in length. Although generally found on the pubic hairs, the crab louse attaches to hair on other parts of the body, such as the scalp or axilla. **Pediculosis ciliaris**, seen mostly in children, is due to pubic louse infestation of the eyelids.

Pediculosis corporis is caused by a larger louse that feeds on the skin but does not remain attached to it, preferring to reside in the seams of clothing. Intense itching leads to eczematization—**vagabonds' disease.** Body lice can transmit epidemic typhus (*Rickettsia prowazekii*), trench fever (*Bartonella quintana*), and louse-borne relapsing fever (*Borrelia recurrentis*).

Figure 5–1　Pediculosis capitis with clearly visible nits.

DIFFERENTIAL DIAGNOSIS

Seborrheic dermatitis—"walking dandruff"—is scaling, and the scales do not stick to the hair. It can be distinguished by its successful treatment with tar shampoo. Contact dermatitis and drug eruptions cause diffuse pruritus.

HOW TO MAKE THE DIAGNOSIS

Finding the live louse or nit on a hair shaft makes the diagnosis of head louse and pubic louse infestation. A hand lens is helpful in identifying the nit, which is attached to the hair shaft by a cementum (Fig. 5–2). Wood's light examination shows whitish fluorescence of the hair and the nits. Inspection of the patient's clothing, particularly the seams, will reveal body lice. Often, these diagnostic features are absent, and a presumptive diagnosis is made on the basis of excoriations in typical areas.

TREATMENT

Both head lice and crab lice infestations can be treated with 5% permethrin or 1% lindane shampoo, which is applied for 10 minutes and rinsed off; this is repeated in a day or a week. (Lindane should not be used on infants or pregnant women.) The nits can remain. Combing them out can be assisted by using white vinegar while rinsing.

Body lice infestation is managed by washing the clothes in hot water or disposing of them. The skin is then treated symptomatically with corticosteroid

Figure 5–2 Nit attached to hair shaft seen with a hand lens.

ointments or creams. The strength of these preparations depends on the degree of itch; usually, medium-potent to high-potent creams are needed. Insecticides are not needed. Although nits can live off the skin for 1 or 2 days, they are sensitive enough to the temperature changes of daily living, hence additional treatment is not necessary. Nits can transmit infestation in close contact, therefore, treatment of household members and schoolmates is recommended.

PROGNOSIS

Treatment failure is due to inadequate shampooing or reinfestation.

Chapter 6

DYSHIDROTIC ECZEMA
(ICD-9 705.81)

Lawrence Charles Parish

SYMPTOMS AND SIGNS

Patients with dyshidrotic eczema complain of itching or burning, which is sometimes intense. The hallmark of dyshidrotic eczema is deep-seated, clear blisters on the sides of the fingers (Fig. 6–1) and on the palms and soles. Because the epidermis is thicker in these areas, the blisters are deep and are often said to look like tapioca pudding. When they break, collarettes of scale are left behind that last 2 to 3 weeks. Sometimes, there is oozing and crusting. Dyshidrotic eczema may be associated with hyperhidrosis, atopic dermatitis, or contact dermatitis. Symptoms are worse in warm weather, but the condition may flare in winter if the skin is dry. The disease is also called **pompholyx**.

DIFFERENTIAL DIAGNOSIS

Atopic dermatitis and contact dermatitis are usually not limited to the sides of the fingers, although they can be present on only the palms or soles. Rarely,

Figure 6–1 Pruritic vesicles on the sides of the fingers.

id reactions to dermatophytes or bacteria mimic dyshidrosis; however, tinea pedis and tinea manuum are more disseminated on the feet or hands and are often more erythematous.

HOW TO MAKE THE DIAGNOSIS

The clinical presentation of dyshidrotic eczema suggests the diagnosis. Look especially for tapioca pudding-like vesicles.

TREATMENT

Medium-potent to super-potent topical corticosteroid creams or ointments can control acute conditions. Secondary bacterial infection may require oral erythromycin or cephalexin, 250 mg three to four times daily for 7 to 10 days. For weeping lesions, compresses of Burow's solution in water (1:40) are applied for 5 minutes three times daily. Addition of ice water to dilute the powder offers more relief. After the acute outbreak is relieved, a low-potent topical corticosteroid may be used to suppress the condition.

PROGNOSIS

Dyshidrosis shows waxing and waning. Usually, acute attacks clear within 1 or 2 weeks of treatment, but occasionally, it smolders for months.

Chapter 7

STASIS DERMATITIS
(ICD-9 454.1)

Lawrence Charles Parish

SYMPTOMS AND SIGNS

Stasis dermatitis may initially cause an aching or gnawing feeling in the legs. Itching and burning are often intense enough to lead to excoriations, secondary bacterial infection, and even an **id reaction**, which is dermatitis that appears at a distant site on the body, usually the hands and arms. Stasis dermatitis usually occurs in older patients when venous or lymphatic return to the legs has been compromised. With increased extravasation of blood into the tissues, darkening becomes more permanent, and soon erythema, scaling, and oozing appear (Fig. 7–1). Occasionally, the process leads to irregularly shaped ulcerations known as **stasis ulcers** (see Chapter 70).

DIFFERENTIAL DIAGNOSIS

Stasis dermatitis is limited to the legs, but the eruption can mimic that of contact dermatitis and neurodermatitis. The former was common in the past

Figure 7–1   Stasis dermatitis causes erythema, scaling, and sometimes oozing on the lower legs.

with the use of topical anesthetics and ammoniated mercury; the latter is distinguished by patches of dermatitis being found elsewhere on the body.

HOW TO MAKE THE DIAGNOSIS

Patchy redness and scaling on the legs constitute the hallmark of stasis dermatitis until proved otherwise.

TREATMENT

High-potent or super-potent topical corticosteroid cream or ointment, applied twice daily for several weeks or months, is needed to resolve the acute inflammation. Secondary infection can be treated with erythromycin, 250 mg three times daily by mouth for 7 to 10 days. Patients should also elevate their legs and wear support hosiery.

PROGNOSIS

Stasis dermatitis is a chronic condition that smolders for years. With appropriate therapy, it can be controlled.

Chapter 8

PRURITUS AND EXCORIATIONS WITH NO PRIMARY SKIN LESIONS
(Generalized Pruritus ICD-9 698.9;
Lichen Simplex Chronicus ICD-9 698.3;
Prurigo Nodularis ICD-9 698.3)

Jeffrey P. Callen

SYMPTOMS AND SIGNS

Many patients complain of pruritus but have either no discernible rash or a rash that is initiated by scratching.

One of the more common causes of pruritus is dry skin, particularly in the elderly and during winter. It is worsened with bathing and/or using harsh soaps. Patients may have no visible skin changes, or they may develop excoriated, eczematous patches, which can become impetiginized.

When no visible changes are present, an attempt should be made to elicit **dermatographism**, the appearance of a hive from stroking of the skin (Fig. 15–2). Dermatographism is more common in patients with urticaria.

Patients without obvious skin diseases should also be evaluated for systemic disease. Common causes are renal disease (uremia and hemodialysis-related), hepatobiliary disease (primary biliary cirrhosis and cholestatic problems), thyroid disease (both hypothyroidism and hyperthyroidism), diabetes mellitus, hematologic disease (polycythemia vera), malignancy (lymphoma), and human immunodeficiency virus (HIV) infection.

Drugs associated with pruritus include antibiotics, opiates, bleomycin, angiotensin-converting enzyme inhibitors, diuretics, sulfonylureas, estrogens, antithyroid agents, and anticoagulants.

Two conditions initiated by constant scratching are **prurigo nodularis** and **lichen simplex chronicus**. Large, firm, hyperpigmented nodules of prurigo nodularis often develop in crops on the arms and legs (Fig. 8–1). Lichen simplex chronicus involves intense itching and habitual scratching the skin of a particular area. Lichenification is the hallmark sign, but the lesions are also notably red and scaling. Common sites are the lower legs, neck, wrists, and ankles (Fig. 8–2).

DIFFERENTIAL DIAGNOSIS

In patients with excoriations, causes such as scabies, eczemas, or dermatitis herpetiformis should be excluded. Patients with scabies have intense nocturnal pruritus and excoriations with burrows on the wrists, genitalia, and web spaces of the hands, and their family members have similar symptoms. Dermatitis herpetiformis manifests as symmetric grouped excoriations, and occasionally vesicles, on extensor surfaces such as the elbows or buttocks. Eczemas have typical distribution patterns and eventual lichenification.

HOW TO MAKE THE DIAGNOSIS

Scabies can be confirmed by skin scrapings. Patients with findings suggestive of dermatitis herpetiformis should undergo a punch biopsy of lesional skin for

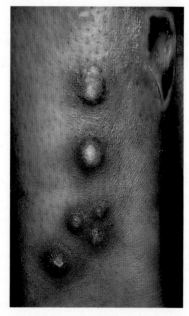

Figure 8–1 Prurigo nodularis, with multiple pruritic, hyperpigmented nodules on the arms also demonstrates a self-induced ulcer.

Figure 8–2 Lichen simplex chronicus involves intense itching and habitual scratching of the skin of a particular area (the shin, in this patient).

routine processing and of perilesional normal-appearing skin for immunofluorescence microscopy. The presence of systemic disease in patients is often evident by history. However, at a minimum, patients should have a physical examination and a complete blood count; liver, renal, and thyroid function tests; a hepatitis C antibody test; and a chest x-ray.

TREATMENT

General care of the patient with generalized pruritus involves application of emollients. Occasionally, a medium-potent corticosteroid cream or ointment is helpful for temporary relief. But if the itch is generalized, topical corticosteroids are impractical and can result in corticosteroid-related systemic toxicity from percutaneous absorption. Lotions containing 0.25% to 0.5% menthol or phenol, or 0.25% menthol in a medium-potency corticosteroid cream, may give temporary relief. Oral antihistamines such as hydroxyzine 10 to 25 mg, cyproheptadine 4 mg, or doxepin 25 to 50 mg, should be taken before sleep and three to four times daily, as needed. Nonsedating and mildly sedating antihistamines offer little benefit. Topical antihistamines are not recommended because they may cause contact dermatitis.

Pruritus due to an underlying systemic disease may cease once the underlying disease is successfully treated. For patients with renal disease, hepatobiliary disease, and HIV-associated pruritus, medically supervised ultraviolet B phototherapy may be helpful. Malignancy-associated pruritus abates with remission and reappears with relapse.

Prurigo nodularis and lichen simplex chronicus require high-potent to super-potent topical corticosteroid cream or ointment and encouraging, supportive care. These lesions can be stubborn.

PROGNOSIS

Prognosis depends on the cause. In idiopathic disease, there are no life-threatening consequences of generalized pruritus.

Chapter 9

ACNE VULGARIS
(ICD-9 706.1)

James C. Shaw

SYMPTOMS AND SIGNS

Acne vulgaris is usually asymptomatic, although the large nodular lesions can be tender. Patients usually present during adolescence with comedones, papules, pustules, nodules, or a combination of these. Closed comedones (whiteheads) and open comedones (blackheads) represent keratin-plugged hair follicles. The dark color is due to oxidation of surface keratin. Papules and pustules are 2 to 4 mm in diameter and have a slightly erythematous base (Fig. 9–1).

The nodules are deeper, erythematous lesions ranging from 6 to 20 mm in diameter (Fig. 9–2) and occur on the face, neck, back, and chest. The term "cystic acne" is inaccurate and has been replaced by "severe nodular acne" as the preferred nomenclature. Acne is not limited to adolescence and commonly manifests for the first time in adulthood, especially in women.

DIFFERENTIAL DIAGNOSIS

Due to chemical exposures (aromatic chlorinated hydrocarbons such as dioxin and herbicides), comedones cause extensive face and neck lesions. Papules and pustules can be seen in rosacea, bacterial folliculitis, or "steroid acne" that is caused by systemic or topical corticosteroids. A culture of the papules may be required to exclude bacterial folliculitis.

Figure 9–1 Acne vulgaris. Inflammatory papules and pustules.

Figure 9–2 Nodular acne is the main indication for isotretinoin therapy.

HOW TO MAKE THE DIAGNOSIS

Acne vulgaris is a clinical diagnosis. The presence of open or closed comedones in an adolescent patient is usually confirmatory for acne vulgaris. If a patient presents with only pustules on the face, a bacterial culture may be required to exclude bacterial folliculitis.

TREATMENT

Patients must be told at the beginning of therapy that response to any treatment may take up to 6 weeks and that patience on their part (and on their doctor's part) will usually be rewarded. In general, it is helpful to advise patients having acne that gentle washing once or twice daily is sufficient. Scrubs, abrasives, and alcohol-based toners/clarifiers are often irritating, especially when combined with topical acne medications that can dry and inflame the skin. Washing does not cure acne. It merely washes off oils, dirt, makeup, and so on.

For patients with only comedonal disease, topical comedolytic agents are appropriate; tretinoin 0.01% to 0.05%, adapalene 0.1%, or tazarotene 0.1% applied nightly on the dry skin is effective. Tretinoin comes in several strengths. Creams are better tolerated than gels, but less effective. Adapalene is better tolerated than tretinoin, while tazarotene, though shown to be more effective, causes more irritation. Keratolytic agents are generally applied once daily but can be used twice daily if tolerated. Sunscreens may prevent sun sensitivity caused by any of these agents.

Patients with superficial inflammatory papules require topical antimicrobial agents. These may be combined with comedolytics. Benzoyl peroxide—containing gels, creams, or washes should be applied once daily. Start with a 5% gel or cream in the morning. Decrease to 2.5% if this is too irritating or increase to 10%, as needed. Washes are best for large areas such as the back and chest. Clindamycin 1% or erythromycin 2% in combination with benzoyl peroxide is more effective than either product alone. Combination products are available as gels, creams, or pledgets. Azelaic acid 20%, an antibacterial and comedolytic, has been shown to be effective and well tolerated.

For moderately severe inflammatory acne, systemic antibiotics must be used for at least 1 to 3 months. Choices and dosages include tetracycline 500 mg twice daily, doxycycline 50 to 100 mg twice daily, minocycline 100 to 200 mg daily, erythromycin 250 mg four times daily, or erythromycin ethylsuccinate 400 mg two to three times daily.

In patients with severe nodular acne, in recalcitrant cases, or when there is scarring, isotretinoin is the drug of choice. The standard dosing is 1 to 2 mg/kg daily for 4 to 6 months. Experience with use of isotretinoin and knowledge of its complications is essential for safe use. This drug is contraindicated in women of childbearing age without adequate birth control measures and counseling. Two forms of contraception are recommended for women taking this drug who do not choose abstinence.

Pretreatment blood workup includes two pregnancy tests, complete blood count, liver function studies, and lipid profile. These tests should be repeated monthly. Common side effects are cheilitis (90%) and elevated serum triglyceride levels (25%). The less common ones are conjunctivitis, xerosis, musculoskeletal pains, arthralgias, and hair thinning. Cheilitis is best treated with an ointment such as petroleum jelly. It is often helpful to advise patients to put petroleum jelly inside the nose at bedtime to prevent bleeding from a dry nasal mucosa. Sunscreens should be used daily because of photosensitivity. Depression has never been proven to be caused by isotretinoin, but patients should be advised of the potential relationship and monitored.

Acne in women sometimes presents special considerations, including hormonal causes and the possibility of polycystic ovary syndrome. Hormonal therapies can be effective in any woman with acne. Oral contraceptives, androgen receptor blockers, and insulin sensitizers have all had success, although only select oral contraceptives are U.S. Food and Drug Administration (FDA) approved for acne.

PROGNOSIS

Most patients with adolescent acne improve spontaneously. Nonetheless, there may be severe and lifelong psychological effects. Patients with adult acne can continue to have episodic or persistent involvement for many years.

Chapter 10

PERIORAL DERMATITIS
(ICD-695.3)

Jeffrey P. Callen

SIGNS AND SYMPTOMS

Although lesions of perioral dermatitis may burn or feel tender, most patients complain about their appearance rather than about specific symptoms. The disease is more common in women and usually occurs in early adulthood (25 to 35 years of age). Erythematous papules and pustules with minimal scales are the characteristic lesions (Fig. 10–1). This condition may be worsened by fluorinated topical corticosteroids or by fluorinated tartar control toothpastes.

DIFFERENTIAL DIAGNOSIS

Rosacea has more extensive facial lesions and greater amounts of flushing. Acne vulgaris has other types of lesions such as comedos and larger cysts, and the patients are often younger. Contact dermatitis is pruritic and can often be linked to a specific agent. Seborrhea is scaly, is located on the central face, and has accompanying dandruff.

HOW TO MAKE THE DIAGNOSIS

The diagnosis is made by clinical examination. Punch biopsy or laboratory testing is rarely necessary. Patch testing excludes a contact dermatitis.

TREATMENT

A low-potent topical corticosteroid cream or ointment compounded with 1% precipitated sulfur is helpful. Alternatives include metronidazole 0.075%

Figure 10–1 Perioral dermatitis. Erythematous perioral papules seen almost exclusively in young women.

cream or gel, and topical clindamycin 2% or erythromycin 2% in lotions, gels, or foams. Topical products that contain sulfacetamide with or without sulfur might also be useful. Topical azelaic acid preparations might also be considered, but irritation may limit their use. Oral tetracycline, 500 to 1,000 mg daily, is also helpful. The onset of effect, however, is delayed by 4 to 6 weeks. Recalcitrant individual lesions may be injected with small amounts (<0.05 mL) of triamcinolone acetonide solution in a concentration of 3 mg/mL.

PROGNOSIS

Perioral dermatitis heals spontaneously, but this may take years to occur.

Chapter 11

ROSACEA
(ICD-9 695.3)

Larry E. Millikan

SYMPTOMS AND SIGNS

The classic symptom of rosacea is flushing, although this is often lacking. Patients usually complain of a red nose or face. The condition is made worse by hot (temperature) or spicy foods or beverages, alcohol, and sunlight. The findings can be subtle and merely limited to mild telangiectasia and centrofacial erythema. More pronounced rosacea appears as acneiform facial papules, pustules, and frank ruddiness (Fig. 11–1). Some clinicians talk of the "rosacea oval," a vertical pattern of erythema from the glabella to the chin. Thickening and enlargement of nasal skin can cause the characteristic bulbous nose of rhinophyma, but this is rare. Northern European and Celtic patients are affected most. Eye diseases, such as conjunctivitis, blepharitis, episcleritis, or keratitis, are common complications of rosacea.

DIFFERENTIAL DIAGNOSIS

Erythema from seborrheic dermatitis is accompanied by scaling on the scalp, nasal creases, and nasolabial folds. Acne vulgaris is not as often centrofacial or telangiectatic. Contact dermatitis will have a suggestive history and itching. Skin changes of systemic lupus erythematosus are malar and induced by sunlight.

Figure 11–1   Rosacea. This woman has "rosy cheeks" and telangiectasias with inflammatory papules and pustules.

HOW TO MAKE DIAGNOSIS

History—especially the relationship to certain foods—genetic tendency, and centrofacial involvement are usually sufficient to make the diagnosis of rosacea.

TREATMENT

The traditional oral treatment is tetracycline, 500 mg twice daily; doxycycline, 100 mg twice daily, is an alternative. Metronidazole 0.075% gel or cream two to three times daily is often effective but may take several months to work; 15% azelaic acid gel daily is also effective. Rhinophyma can be treated by laser or electrosurgery. Eye symptoms should be evaluated by an ophthalmologist.

PROGNOSIS

Treatment usually provides symptomatic relief. It is not clear if early aggressive therapy impedes the rare progression to rhinophyma.

Chapter 12

SEBORRHEIC DERMATITIS
(ICD-9 609.1)

Larry E. Millikan

SYMPTOMS AND SIGNS

Seborrheic dermatitis (SD) of the face is often pruritic, but only mildly so. Itching of the scalp, however, is a common symptom. There is erythema and fine, bran-like scaling on the forehead, nasolabial folds, around the ears, and on the eyebrows or eyelids (Fig. 12–1). The scalp is often involved—common dandruff—as are presternal and intertriginous areas, such as the vault of the axilla and the groin. Seborrheic blepharitis is SD of the eyelids and margins. The condition can be florid in patients with acquired immunodeficiency syndrome (AIDS).

DIFFERENTIAL DIAGNOSIS

Psoriasis has a typical pattern of distribution on the elbows, knees, scalp, and nails. In tinea, lesions are more circumscribed and hyphae are seen under the microscope. The hallmark of candidiasis is intertriginous involvement. Contact dermatitis can be distinguished by the history of the offending agent and more pruritus. Patients with rosacea have a history of flushing, and the centrofacial erythema is not accompanied by scales.

HOW TO MAKE THE DIAGNOSIS

Diagnosis of SD is made on clinical distribution and response to therapy. It is worthwhile to look for evidence of SD in all possible body sites.

Figure 12–1 Seborrheic dermatitis. Erythema and fine, bran-like scaling on eyebrows.

33

TREATMENT

SD is a chronic and recurring condition, and patients may treat themselves without supervision for long periods. Therefore, use only low-potent topical corticosteroid ointments or creams. Antifungal creams of the imidazole or allylamine classes can also be effective but work more slowly. High-potent or super-potent corticosteroid solutions are safe on the scalp for long periods. Medicated shampoos should contain tar, zinc, sulfur, or salicylic acid. The antifungal shampoo, ketoconazole 2%, can be used twice weekly. "Off-label" tacrolimus and pimecrolimus have been reported as effective. Recent change in labeling "Black Box" should be considered in this "Off-label" usage.

PROGNOSIS

SD often recurs in times of stress, either physical or emotional. Seborrheic blepharitis can lead to recurring infections of the eyelids, with hordeolum and conjunctivitis.

Chapter 13

LUPUS ERYTHEMATOSUS
(ICD-9 695.4)

Jeffrey P. Callen

SIGNS AND SYMPTOMS

Cutaneous lupus erythematosus (LE) can be divided into chronic, subacute, and acute forms. Patients may complain of photosensitivity, mildly pruritic or painful skin lesions, and/or arthralgias.

Chronic cutaneous LE is most commonly manifest as **discoid lupus erythematosus** (DLE). Lesions of DLE are red with adherent scale, telangiectasia, follicular plugging, and dyspigmentation. Atrophy and scarring are characteristic (Fig. 13–1). Lesions most often occur on the head, neck, ears, scalp, arms, and upper chest and back. Less than 5% of patients with DLE have systemic manifestations of lupus.

Systemic lupus erythematosus (SLE) often presents as the classic, malar "butterfly" rash when the skin is involved (Fig. 13–2). The rash is exacerbated by sun exposure or exposure to ultraviolet B (UVB) or ultraviolet A (UVA) from artificial light sources. Almost all patients with a butterfly rash have active SLE. **Subacute cutaneous lupus erythematosus** (SCLE) lesions are of at least two types: annular or papulosquamous. Both forms begin as red papules or plaques on sun-exposed skin, which eventually expand and form either rings or psoriasiform lesions. Annular lesions have central clearing. Papulosquamous lesions are scaling. Approximately 50% of patients with

Figure 13–1 Discoid lupus erythematosus with sharply marginated atrophic plaques with patulous follicles.

Figure 13-2   Subacute cutaneous lupus erythematosus with characteristic annular lesions.

SCLE have evidence of systemic manifestations of lupus. SCLE is associated with Sjögren's syndrome, idiopathic thrombocytopenic purpura, cutaneous vasculitis, or deficiency of the second component of complement (C2d). It may be induced by a variety of drugs, most commonly hydrochlorothiazide, other antihypertensive agents, and terbinafine.

DIFFERENTIAL DIAGNOSIS

DLE and papulosquamous SCLE may simulate many other papulosquamous disorders. Psoriasis often has the classic knee, elbow, and scalp distribution. Lichen planus papules are violaceous, and oral lesions are common. Secondary syphilis involves the palms and soles. Dermatophytes do not preferentially infect sun-exposed skin, and papules of sarcoidosis are waxy, translucent, and without scale. Annular SCLE must be differentiated from dermatophyte infection and figurate erythemas. The malar rash of SLE may be confused with rosacea or seborrheic dermatitis.

HOW TO MAKE THE DIAGNOSIS

Punch biopsy usually confirms the diagnosis. Rarely, an additional biopsy specially processed for immunofluorescence microscopy is needed to confirm the diagnosis in patients with scarring alopecia or mucosal disease. The antinuclear antibody (ANA) is a nonspecific test. It is almost always positive in SCLE and SLE, but only in 15% to 30% of patients with DLE. The anti-Ro (SS-A) antibody is frequently positive in patients with SCLE; however, it should not be used to confirm or rule out the diagnosis. Antinative (double-stranded) deoxyribonucleic acid (DNA) is specific for SLE, particularly renal disease.

TREATMENT

Photosensitivity is a major factor in all types of cutaneous LE. Therefore sunscreens that block UVA and UVB and sun avoidance are a cornerstone of therapy. Sunscreens must be used everyday. Topical corticosteroids should be prescribed in conjunction with other agents. The strength is based on the clinical lesion and area of the body that is affected. Lesions that do not respond to topical agents can be injected intralesionally with minute amounts (less than 0.05 mL) of triamcinolone acetonide suspension in a concentration of 3 mg/mL.

Antimalarial agents are the mainstay of systemic therapy for cutaneous LE. The oral agents available include hydroxychloroquine, 200 to 400 mg daily, and chloroquine phosphate, 250 to 500 mg daily; however, the daily dose should be kept below 6.5 mg/kg per day and 4 mg/kg per day respectively. Both agents may cause retinopathy. Ophthalmologic examination and periodic reevaluation are necessary. Patients who fail to respond or who develop toxicity to the antimalarial agents are often effectively treated with thalidomide. This agent is a potent teratogen and may cause neuropathy and must be carefully monitored.

Chapter 14

DERMATOMYOSITIS
(ICD-9 710.3)

Jeffrey P. Callen

SYMPTOMS AND SIGNS

Skin lesions of dermatomyositis (DM) are often pruritic. The characteristic lesions are the heliotrope rash and Gottron's papules. The heliotrope rash consists of a periorbital violaceous to dusky erythematous rash, which may be edematous (Fig. 14–1). Gottron's papules are erythematosus to violaceous papules or plaques found over bony prominences, particularly over the metacarpophalangeal joints, the proximal interphalangeal joints, and the distal interphalangeal joints (Fig. 14–2). Nail-fold changes consist of periungual telangiectasias and cuticular hypertrophy with small hemorrhagic infarcts. Patches of poikiloderma—mottled, atrophic, and telangiectatic skin—develop on exposed surfaces, such as the extensor arm and the anterior V of the neck. The scalp may be red and intensely pruritic with diffuse scale and alopecia. Calcinosis of the skin or muscle is unusual in adults but may occur in up to 40% of children with DM, particularly those who are not treated aggressively with corticosteroids and/or immunosuppressive agents.

More than 90% of patients with skin lesions eventually have myopathy, but the skin lesions may precede muscle disease by months to years. There are a small group of patients who never develop weakness and in whom repeated muscle enzyme testing is normal; these patients are said to have amyopathic DM. The myopathy of DM mainly affects the proximal muscle groups of

Figure 14–1 Dermatomyositis. Periorbital lilac discoloration of heliotrope rash.

Figure 14–2 Gottron's papules are flat-topped erythematous papules and plaques over bony prominences on the dorsal hands.

the shoulder and pelvic girdles and is usually symmetric. Initial complaints include weakness, fatigue, inability to climb stairs and raise the arms for hair grooming or shaving, and weakness in rising from a squatting or sitting position. Arthralgias or arthritis occur in up to 25% of patients. Dysphagia is present in 20% to 50% and can be either proximal or distal. Approximately 20% of patients with DM have an associated malignancy regardless of whether or not they have myositis. Malignancy usually appears within the first 3 years following diagnosis.

DIFFERENTIAL DIAGNOSIS

The skin lesions of DM are often difficult to differentiate from lupus erythematosus, but patients with DM have more cuticular changes and more intense pruritus. Psoriasis, lichen planus, and chronic eczemas may also be considered until the classic features of DM appear. Punch biopsy can exclude all these conditions except lupus erythematosus.

HOW TO MAKE THE DIAGNOSIS

The heliotrope rash and Gottron's papules are the most helpful signs, but they are not always present in patients with DM. Laboratory testing includes serum creatine kinase or aldolase or both. An electromyogram, muscle biopsy, or magnetic resonance imaging (MRI) of the muscles may be necessary. Once a diagnosis is established the patient should be assessed with a complete physical examination, a barium swallow, a chest x-ray and pulmonary function tests, an electrocardiogram, and tests to exclude a potential malignancy.

TREATMENT

The mainstay of therapy for myositis is systemic corticosteroids. Prednisone, 0.5 to 1 mg/kg daily by mouth, is the initial therapy. Immunosuppressive agents including methotrexate, azathioprine, cyclophosphamide, chlorambucil, mycophenolate mofetil, sirolimus, or cyclosporine are used in nonresponsive patients or in patients who develop steroid-related toxicity. In patients who fail these therapies, the use of intravenous immunoglobulin 1 gm/kg per day on two consecutive days monthly has been demonstrated to be effective.

Even when the myositis responds to these measures, the skin disease may persist. Hydroxychloroquine, 200 to 400 mg daily by mouth, is effective treatment for skin disease in approximately 80% of patients; however, roughly 20% of patients treated with hydroxychloroquine will develop a drug eruption. For skin disease oral corticosteroids are often used, but are rarely effective; immunosuppressive agents including methotrexate, mycophenolate mofetil, and intravenous immunoglobulin are often helpful in controlling this disabling dermatosis. Finally, patients with DM and cutaneous lesions are exquisitely photosensitive, so sunscreens with a high sun protective factor (SPF) and a broad spectrum should be applied daily.

PROGNOSIS

Prognosis of patients with DM varies, depending on the series reported. Factors predisposing to poor outcome are advanced age, severe myositis, dysphagia, associated malignancy, and poor response to corticosteroid therapy.

Chapter 15

URTICARIA
(ICD-9 708.9)

Larry E. Millikan

SYMPTOMS AND SIGNS

Urticaria is pruritic. The degree of pruritus depends on the amount of swelling. Patients often say they can watch the lesions come and go within hours. The lesions are evanescent and migratory and do not last beyond 24 hours. Urticaria presents as elevated and edematous plaques, usually pale red or pink. As the lesions spread, there is often a central clearing, which leaves an arcuate or gyrate formation (Fig. 15–1).

Urticaria may be acute or chronic. By definition, acute urticaria lasts less than 6 weeks, and chronic urticaria lasts longer. The causes of either are rarely found. Common precipitants include salicylates and penicillins. Salicylates are found in spearmint and wintergreen flavors as in toothpaste, candies, and tomatoes. Penicillins can be found in bleu cheese dressing and some dairy products. Menthol is the culprit in peppermint toothpaste or

Figure 15–1 Urticaria. Central clearing of urticarial lesions leads to arcuate appearance that is sometimes confused with tinea corporis.

41

mentholated cigarettes. Other causes include foods (seafoods, strawberries, FDC Yellow 5), opiates, antibiotics, antiepileptics, and systemic diseases such as lupus erythematosus and paraproteinemias.

Urticaria can also be caused by physical agents, such as heat, cold, ultraviolet light, and the trauma of scratching (dermatographism). Exercise-induced urticaria (cholinergic urticaria) produces small lesions 1 to 2 mm in diameter.

DIFFERENTIAL DIAGNOSIS

Erythema multiforme, urticarial vasculitis, bullous pemphigoid, collagen vascular disease, and mastocytosis may present with widespread urticarial plaques. Atopic eczema and contact dermatitis may also be urticarial, but these are more pruritic. Miliaria and folliculitis resemble cholinergic urticaria. Urticarial lesions with central clearing resemble tinea corporis.

HOW TO MAKE THE DIAGNOSIS

Diagnosis of urticaria can often be made purely on history, symptoms, and signs. Dermatographism can be elicited by lightly scratching the skin (Fig. 15–2). When the diagnosis is not certain, a punch biopsy may help.

TREATMENT

The premise is that histamine is the major physiologic agent inducing urticaria. Since the vasculature has both H_1 and H_2 receptors, it is important to consider the use of both types of antihistamine. The *caveat* with most antihistamines is adequate dosing. Keep in mind that the recommended dosage is usually for a 70-kg patient. In our affluent, well-fed society, many patients are at least 50% over the average weight.

For mild, limited disease, withdrawing the causative agent may be all that is needed. In addition, oral H_1 blockers may be helpful. These include desloratadine 5 mg daily; cetirizine, 10 mg daily; hydroxyzine, 25 mg two to three times daily; or cyproheptadine, 4 mg four times daily. If this is not effective, an H_2 blocker, such as cimetidine, 300 mg daily by mouth, may be

Figure 15–2   Urticaria. Dermatographism elicited after light scratching.

added. Other H_2 blockers can be effective but are more expensive. Finally, a short course of an oral corticosteroid tapered over 10 days may be needed. A good beginning dose is prednisone 1.0 mg/kg daily.

PROGNOSIS

In most patients acute urticaria clears on therapy without the cause being identified. The prognosis in any chronic urticaria is guarded. Patients should always understand that urticaria, acute or chronic, is a serious symptom complex that may not respond to therapy and that oral corticosteroid treatment to prevent serious airway complications may be necessary for prolonged periods.

Chapter 16

ERYTHEMA MULTIFORME
(ICD-9 695.1)

Larry E. Millikan

SYMPTOMS AND SIGNS

We must begin with a note on terminology. There is confusion because the term erythema multiforme (EM) describes a spectrum of disease whose boundaries seem to shift by author. Authors are either "splitters" or "lumpers."

Splitters divide the EM spectrum into several entities, beginning with mild EM and severe EM. Mild EM has mild skin involvement and sometimes mild mucosal involvement, usually the mouth. Severe EM has more advanced skin involvement and prominent mucosal involvement, including the mouth, labia, and conjunctiva. To confuse things further, some splitters label the severe form of EM the Stevens–Johnson syndrome (SJS). Furthermore, toxic epidermal necrolysis (TEN), with its massive skin sloughing, is considered in this scheme to be yet another, separate entity.

Lumpers divide the spectrum into only two groups, EM and TEN/SJS. For this book, we will use the simpler scheme of the lumpers (see Chapter 31).

The symptoms of EM may be minimal—a feeling of warmth or pruritus of involved skin—or severe. Bullous lesions may be very painful. Pain on the palms is a good clue to the diagnosis. The primary sign of EM is erythema; the classic lesions are targets (Fig. 16–1; see also Fig. 31–2). Target (or iris) lesions are round with a central dusky red bull's-eye surrounded by edematous concentric pink rings. EM may also be arcuate like common

Figure 16–1 The primary sign of erythema multiforme is erythema; the classic lesion is the target.

Figure 16–2 Erythema multiforme. Arcuate lesions with central clearing may resemble common urticaria.

urticaria or bullous (Fig. 16–2). The distribution and extent of involvement can be variable. However, EM usually begins as a symmetric eruption on the extensor extremities and may progress to trunk or facial involvement.

DIFFERENTIAL DIAGNOSIS

Although the arcuate rings of urticarial lesions may be indistinguishable from EM, urticarial lesions resolve within 24 hours. Angioedema involves larger areas of skin and is indurated. Early contact dermatitis can usually be ruled out by lack of contact with an offending agent. A final consideration would be graft versus host disease, which occurs only in specific situations.

HOW TO MAKE THE DIAGNOSIS

The patient's history is crucial, especially when the lesions are early and there are no targets. Pain is a key symptom of EM. Check for a history of drug therapy or infection by *Mycoplasma pneumoniae* or herpes simplex. Common drugs that trigger EM are sulfonamides, penicillin, barbiturates, and phenytoin. Remember that at least 50% of patients with EM have a negative history. Punch biopsy may be useful in confirming the clinical diagnosis. Eye symptoms mandate opthalmologic consultation.

TREATMENT

Elimination of a causative drug or infectious agent is most helpful for patients with EM. Pruritus can be treated with antihistamines. More advanced disease may respond to systemic oral corticosteroids such as prednisone, 1.0 mg/kg daily, in the very early phases. In TEN/SJS, the role of systemic corticosteroids is uncertain. Patients with TEN/SJS must be treated in a burn facility. Severe cases may require intravenous immunoglobulin (IVIg) and other biological agents for therapy.

PROGNOSIS

Mild EM in children and adults has an excellent prognosis and usually resolves within 2 to 4 weeks. Sequelae may include postinflammatory pigment changes and scarring. Suppressive treatment of herpes simplex infection may break the cycle of EM recurrence. TEN/SJS is a severe disease, which may progress to death.

Chapter 17

DRUG ERUPTION
(ICD-9 693.0)

Larry E. Millikan

SYMPTOMS AND SIGNS

Symptoms of drug eruption can vary and may include itching, pruritus, burning, or frank skin pain. Symptoms usually correlate with the severity of the reaction. Skin pain is associated with severe reactions and may be a harbinger of toxic epidermal necrolysis (TEN)/Stevens–Johnson syndrome (SJS). Drug reactions vary in their clinical presentation. In most cases, they occur within 3 weeks of beginning therapy. In some instances, such as penicillin eruptions in previously sensitized patients, the reaction can begin within 1 day of administration.

Urticarial and maculopapular eruptions are the most common eruptions (Fig. 17–1). Bullous reactions and erythema multiforme are less common (Figs. 16–1 and 16–2). Fortunately, palpable purpura (cutaneous vasculitis) (Fig. 62–1) and TEN/SJS (Figs. 31–1 to 31–3) are rare. Some of the more common offending drugs are penicillins, cephalosporins, sulfonamides,

Figure 17–1   Urticarial and maculopapular eruption due to ampicillin.

47

phenytoin, phenobarbital, allopurinol, nonsteroidal anti-inflammatory drugs, and gold.

DIFFERENTIAL DIAGNOSIS

Erythema multiforme and TEN/SJS can be caused by other etiologies. Individual urticarial lesions disappear within 24 hours. Eczema is more pruritic, and photosensitivity reactions have the characteristic distribution on exposed skin, usually the forearms, V area of the upper portion of the neck and the face. Viral exanthems may also be considered, although these often have accompanying respiratory or gastrointestinal symptoms.

HOW TO MAKE THE DIAGNOSIS

Diagnosis requires detective work, especially given the number of new medications introduced each year.

TREATMENT

Elimination of the suspect drug is most important. Symptomatic treatments include topical corticosteroid cream or ointment. The recommended strength depends on the degree of reaction and the patient's discomfort. Usually high-potent agents are given at first. Oral prednisone, 1 mg/kg body weight, may be needed to arrest severe reactions. Oral antihistamines may also bring relief. Some choices are cyproheptadine, 4 mg three times daily and 8 mg at night; desloratadine, 5 mg daily; hydroxyzine, 10 mg three to four times daily (if the patient weighs less than 50 kg) or 25 mg three to four times daily (if the patient weighs over 50 kg); and cetirizine, 10 mg daily.

PROGNOSIS

The outcome is usually excellent with early treatment. TEN/SJS is a serious sign that carries significant morbidity and mortality.

Chapter 18

ERYTHEMA MIGRANS/LYME DISEASE
(ICD-9 088.81)

John T. Crissey

SYMPTOMS AND SIGNS

It is convenient to divide the course and manifestations of Lyme disease (LD) into two stages: early (acute) and late (chronic).

In early LD, 80% of patients present with erythema migrans (EM). Most lesions are asymptomatic. Occasionally, the lesions burn or itch. EM is a highly characteristic skin lesion that first appears as a round or oval erythematous macule at the site of the tick bite (Fig. 18–1). A red punctum at the site of the tick attachment may be present at the center of the ring, the "bull's-eye" in a circular target. The incubation period is 1 to 30 days, with an average of 9 days. Any area of the skin can be affected, and lesions can be single or multiple. The lesions expand nearly 1 cm per day to reach a diameter of 10 to 30 cm. Central clearing is common, giving lesions a ring-like configuration. Regional lymphadenitis may be present. Some patients also experience several days of chills, fever, headache, fatigue, and muscle and joint pain. EM clears spontaneously in a few weeks or months.

Late (chronic) manifestations of the infection appear weeks, months, or years after the tick bite and indicate dissemination of the infection. Intermittent arthritis affects the large joints, especially the knees. Central nervous system (CNS) involvement is common and consists of pain and weakness or numbness in arms or legs, fatigue, disturbances in vision, impaired hearing, facial paralysis (Bell's), or the signs and symptoms of meningitis—headaches,

Figure 18–1 Erythema migrans. Round macule with bull's-eye at site of tick bite.

Figure 18–2   Size comparison. **Left to right:** sesame seed, adult tick, poppy seed, nymph stage, larva stage.

fever, stiff neck, and clouded sensorium. Cardiac involvement is less common and usually appears as a symptomatic variable atrioventricular block.

LD is caused by the spirochete, *Borrelia burgdorferi*. The organism is introduced through the bite of any of several small (2 mm) ticks of the genus *Ixodes*, which are natural parasites of deer, mice, and other mammals that inhabit forested areas (Fig. 18–2). Most cases occur in the northeastern and upper Midwestern areas of the United States, as well as in northern California.

DIFFERENTIAL DIAGNOSIS

Cellulitis and reactions to bites of other insects, especially spiders, can mimic EM. Multiple lesions of EM sometimes resemble erythema multiforme. Fibromyalgia, suggested by the arm and leg pains that often occur in CNS involvement in chronic LD, is the most common misdiagnosis. CNS LD can easily be mistaken for multiple sclerosis and other meningeal infections.

HOW TO MAKE THE DIAGNOSIS

The diagnosis of EM/LD is clinical. It is based on a history of exposure to an area where LD is endemic and on the presence of EM. The causative organism can be identified *in situ* in punch biopsy material taken from EM lesions. It can also be cultured on special media, which is however unavailable in most places. Neither method is practical. Two serologic tests for antibodies to *B. burgdorferi* are available, the enzyme-linked immunosorbent assay (ELISA) and Western immunoblot. Results are often negative in early LD, but are more useful in the later stages. The consensus is that both test results must be positive to establish a diagnosis by serologic means. A new test, the PreVue (Wampole) *B. burgdorferi* antibody detection assay, has now been approved. Results are available within an hour, enabling physicians to make a probable diagnosis and institute treatment much more quickly. Positive results must be confirmed by the Western blot.

TREATMENT

Antibiotic choice and dosage schedules remain in a state of flux at present. Health care providers are encouraged to consult the latest literature for the latest developments. For now, doxycycline, tetracycline, amoxicillin, penicillin G, cefuroxime axetil, ceftriaxone, and cefotaximine are all active against *B. burgdorferi*. For early LD, use doxycycline, 100 mg twice daily by mouth for 21 days (amoxicillin, 25 to 50 mg/kg daily for children under 8 years). For arthritis and mild cardiovascular involvement in later stages, extend the latter regimen to 4 weeks. Patients with neurologic involvement are treated with intravenous ceftriaxone sodium, 2 g daily for 14 to 28 days. No current data support the treatment of patients with asymptomatic tick bites from endemic areas.

PROGNOSIS

The outlook for cure in acute LD is uniformly good. Late cases usually respond well, although some are refractory and require retreatment. Damage to joints and CNS may be severe and permanent. Deaths are rare.

Chapter 19

CANDIDOSIS
(ICD-9 112.9)

Lawrence Charles Parish

SYMPTOMS AND SIGNS

Candida infection on the skin can be asymptomatic or pruritic and burning. Previously called **monilial dermatitis**, it is a yeast infection, most often caused by *Candida albicans*, an organism that is a frequent inhabitant of the gut and the vagina. Candidosis is characterized by red papules and macules that may become confluent, leaving isolated or "satellite" papules and macules at the periphery (Fig. 19–1). Occasionally, the areas become raw, eroded, and begin to ooze. It is often found in the intertriginous areas such as the groin, on the perianal region, and under the breasts, particularly in obese patients. *Candida balanitis* and *Candida vulvovaginitis* often ping-pong between partners. The history may reveal that the patient had diarrhea several days before the onset of the dermatitis or that the female partner has had a vaginal discharge. Diabetics are predisposed to candidosis, and the condition can be florid in immunocompromised patients.

Special types of candidosis include oral candidosis or thrush, in which there are white papules or patches inside the mouth or on the tongue. **Pseudoblastomyces interdigitale** presents as red, scaling areas between the fingers, often under a ring. Monilial paronychia causes redness, induration, swelling, and tenderness around the nail.

DIFFERENTIAL DIAGNOSIS

Seborrheic dermatitis may be confused with candidosis, but the lack of satellite lesions points toward the former. Also, seborrheic dermatitis is found in more locations including the scalp, glabella, paranasal area, submentum, sternum,

Figure 19–1 Candidosis. Erythema, scaling, and satellite lesions in the groin.

axillae, umbilicus, and groin. Contact dermatitis might not be symmetric, and the satellite lesions would be missing. A dermatophyte infection might show central clearing and more scaling.

HOW TO MAKE THE DIAGNOSIS

Candidosis is diagnosed by clinical inspection. A positive 10% potassium hydroxide scraping or culture on fungal medium confirms the diagnosis.

TREATMENT

Localized areas on the skin lend themselves to topical treatment with anti-fungal creams of the imidazole or allylamine classes applied daily or twice daily—depending on the agent—for 2 to 3 weeks (Table 23–1). Extensive cutaneous involvement requires an oral agent such as itraconazole, 100 mg daily for 2 to 4 weeks. Thrush can be treated with nystatin suspension, 100,000 U/mL four times daily, or clotrimazole trouche, 10 mg five times daily. Monilial paronychia is treated systemically with itraconazole, or topically with Thymol 4% in absolute alcohol applied four times daily.

PROGNOSIS

Candidosis can be prevented by keeping the areas dry, treating the vulvo-vaginitis, and keeping the diabetes under control.

Chapter 20

PSORIASIS
(ICD-9 696.1)

James C. Shaw

SYMPTOMS AND SIGNS

Psoriasis is usually asymptomatic, although many patients experience some pruritus. The disease affects 1% of the population of the United States and approximately 3% worldwide. It usually begins by the age of 10, although patients may present any time later. The cardinal features of psoriasis are sharply circumscribed, thick plaques of erythematous skin covered with silvery scales (Fig. 20–1). Nail involvement is common and can be the key to confirming a diagnosis. Look for pitting and nail plate dystrophy (Fig. 20–2). Several types of psoriasis exist.

Plaque psoriasis presents as thick, fixed plaques on the extensor elbows, knees, scalp, lower back, sacral area, and scalp. The demarcation between normal and psoriatic skin is sharp. Any area of the body can be affected, but the face is usually spared. One variant, called **inverse psoriasis**, affects intertriginous areas of the groin, intergluteal cleft, axillae, and inframammary areas.

Guttate psoriasis appears as multiple 0.5- to 1.0-cm psoriatic papules, which develop abruptly on the trunk and extremities, frequently associated with a recent streptococcal pharyngitis (Fig. 20–3).

In **pustular psoriasis**, multiple superficial pustules that may coalesce into pustular lakes develop on previously normal skin or on top of typical, preexisting psoriatic plaques. Pustules are usually all over the body, but a variant of pustular psoriasis is limited to the palms and soles.

Figure 20–1 Plaque psoriasis is sharply demarcated from surrounding normal skin.

Figure 20–2   Psoriatic nail pitting with nail plate dystrophy.

Figure 20–3   Guttate psoriasis is associated with streptococcal pharyngitis.

A rare presentation of psoriasis is a total body **erythroderma**. This can be life-threatening owing to fluid and electrolyte disturbances and thermal dysregulation.

Psoriasis in immunosuppressed human immunodeficiency virus (HIV)-infected individuals is often severe. It commonly has features of both pustular psoriasis and Reiter's syndrome.

Psoriatic arthritis can be present in up to 30% of psoriatics. It usually develops by the age of 30 to 40 years and commonly affects the fingers (polyarticular type) or knees, ankles, and metatarsophalangeal joints (oligoarticular type). Severity of joint disease does not necessarily correlate with the severity of the skin disease.

Several drugs can exacerbate psoriasis, including β-blockers, angiotensin-converting enzyme inhibitors, calcium channel blockers, antimalarials, and interferon.

DIFFERENTIAL DIAGNOSIS

All papulosquamous diseases are included in the differential diagnosis. Pityriasis rosea can resemble guttate psoriasis but the herald patch and Christmas tree distribution are distinguishing features. In discoid lupus erythematosus, thick plaques look like psoriasis, and biopsy may be required to make the distinction. In subacute cutaneous lupus erythematosus, plaques are usually thinner than in typical psoriasis. Unlike psoriasis, both forms of cutaneous lupus are exacerbated by sunlight and often appear on sun-exposed skin. Lichen planus is violaceous and less scaling.

HOW TO MAKE THE DIAGNOSIS

Correct diagnosis of psoriasis is usually made by physical examination. Punch biopsy can be diagnostic in difficult cases. A careful examination of the scalp, umbilicus, intergluteal cleft, and nails can provide clues.

TREATMENT

For limited disease (less than 20% of the body), emollient creams and ointments, and moderate to super-potent topical corticosteroid ointments and creams are the mainstay of therapy. Because psoriasis is a chronic condition, the strength of topical corticosteroid should be reduced as soon as possible to avoid side effects. Calcipotriene 0.005% cream, ointment, or solution twice daily in combination with intermittent topical corticosteroids is usually effective. A topical retinoid, tazarotene gel 0.05% to 0.1% once daily is also an alternative to topical corticosteroids.

For moderate disease (greater than 20% of the body), ultraviolet (UV) light treatments either with ultraviolet B (UVB) or the combination of ultraviolet A (UVA) plus oral psoralens ultraviolet light of A wavelength (PUVA) are frequently effective. Narrow-band UVB (311 nm) has been gaining popularity as a highly effective UV therapy with reduced total accumulative dose.

Widespread disease, pustular psoriasis, and severe psoriatic arthritis require systemic therapies. Methotrexate, systemic retinoid (acetretin), and cyclosporin A are used alone or in combination. A new class of antipsoriasis drugs, the biologic immune response modifiers, has huge promise. Inhibitors of tumor necrosis factor (TNF) (e.g., infliximab, etanercept, adalimumab), and receptor modifiers alefacept and efalizumab are being studied and approved for use in psoriasis. All are delivered parenterally and are expensive, but are a welcomed alternative to existing systemic therapies.

PROGNOSIS

Psoriasis is usually a lifelong disease. Patients may enjoy periods of improvement, but most rely on maintenance treatment to control disease. Morbidity can be significant in patients with psoriatic arthritis and pustular forms. In most cases, there are no medical complications.

Chapter 21

PITYRIASIS ROSEA
(ICD-9 696.3)

Larry E. Millikan

SYMPTOMS AND SIGNS

Pruritus in pityriasis rosea (PR) is usually absent or mild. Rarely is it severe in the papular form of the disease. Many patients recall a "herald patch" as the first sign of PR. The herald patch is red, scaling, and often on the trunk, measuring up to 6 to 7 cm in diameter (Fig. 21–1). Up to 3 weeks later, smaller ovoid macules, 1 to 3 cm in diameter, appear on the trunk and proximal extremities. These lesions sometimes follow a dermatomal distribution on the back, giving the famous "Christmas tree" pattern of PR. But this pattern is not always present. It is far more useful to find lesions with a central collarette of scale, which is a more reliable finding that can make the diagnosis (Fig. 21–2). A rare inverse form of PR causes lesions on the palms, soles, and face.

DIFFERENTIAL DIAGNOSIS

Patients with secondary syphilis have lymphadenopathy. Tinea corporis, psoriasis, and eczema are other considerations, especially when there is a herald patch. In tinea, microscopic examination of scales will show hyphae. Psoriatic lesions, more scaling, and the typical distribution of knees, elbows, nails, and scalp are unlike PR. Eczema is far more pruritic.

HOW TO MAKE THE DIAGNOSIS

The diagnosis of PR is clinical, based on history, herald patch followed by typical lesions and distribution, and general well-being of the patient.

TREATMENT

Treatment of PR depends on the symptoms but is frequently not necessary. Low-potent topical corticosteroid ointment or cream can reduce itching as

Figure 21–1 Pityriasis rosea. The herald patch is easily confused with psoriasis or eczema.

Figure 21–2   Pityriasis rosea. The same patient with typical ovoid lesions showing collarettes of scale.

can creams containing lidocaine or doxepin. Another approach is compounding 1/4% to 1/2% menthol—with or without 1/4% to 1/2% phenol—in moisturizing lotion or cream. Ultraviolet light from the sun is helpful early in the course of disease.

PROGNOSIS

PR is a benign condition and resolves in 2 to 3 months. It recurs in approximately 10% of patients.

Chapter 22

LICHEN PLANUS
(ICD-9 697.0)

Larry E. Millikan

SYMPTOMS AND SIGNS

Lichen planus (LP) can be very pruritic. The classic signs are scaling and purple-to-brown polygonal papules on the wrists, forearms, and legs (Fig. 22–1). The papules are flat on top. A white, shiny, lacy pattern, called **Wickham's striae**, can sometimes be seen on the surface of the papules after application of a drop of oil. A hand lens may be needed to detect this. Approximately two thirds of patients with LP have reticular, white patches or plaques on the buccal mucosa (Fig. 22–2). The head of the penis may also be affected. Hypertrophic LP is a variant, in which thick, large plaques appear on the distal extremities, particularly on the shins. LP of the nails may cause obliteration of the nail fold (pterygium), longitudinal ridging, and pitting.

DIFFERENTIAL DIAGNOSIS

Few other papulosquamous disorders are as pruritic as LP. Guttate psoriasis usually has other lesions that are classic for psoriasis and never has Wickham's striae or mouth lesions. Lichenoid drug eruptions can mimic LP; lesions due to drugs may be identical clinically and histologically. Drugs most likely to cause an LP-like eruption are gold, chloroquine, quinacrine, quinine, tetracycline, griseofulvin, dapsone, penicillamine, and β-blockers.

Patients with very limited early forms of tinea corporis may present with perifollicular papules, but these papules are rarely pruritic and hyphae can be found by microscope examination of scales.

Figure 22–1 Lichen planus. Flat-topped, purple, polygonal papules with shiny, lacy pattern of Wickham's striae.

Figure 22-2 Lichen planus. White, reticular pattern on the buccal mucosa is often a key to the diagnosis.

HOW TO MAKE THE DIAGNOSIS

Diagnosis of LP is established by careful examination. Lesions on the buccal mucosa are helpful. Patients should be tested for hepatitis C, since LP has been associated with this infection. The history may reveal offending drugs. Punch biopsy of a typical lesion usually confirms the diagnosis.

THERAPY

Therapy for LP often requires a trial of different agents. High-potent or super-potent topical corticosteroid ointments or creams seem to be the most consistently effective treatment. Longstanding extensive LP may respond to retinoids or dapsone. Mucous membrane lesions may be treated with potent topical corticosteroids or intralesional injections of triamcinolone acetonide suspension in concentrations of 2.5 to 10 mg/mL to a maximum of 10 to 15 mg weekly.

PROGNOSIS

Most patients with LP heal within 1 year, often with some degree of postinflammatory hyperpigmentation. Recurrences occur in less than 50% of patients.

Chapter 23

TINEA
(ICD-9 110.0 CAPITIS; 110.2 MANUUM;
110.3 CRURIS; 110.4 PEDIS; 110.5 CORPORIS)

Lawrence Charles Parish

SYMPTOMS AND SIGNS

Superficial fungal infections may be asymptomatic, pruritic, or burning. They are often referred to as "ringworm" because the characteristic lesion is a round, scaling, red area with central clearing and sharp, elevated borders. Most dermatophyte infections are caused by species of *Trichophyton, Epidermophyton,* or *Microsporon.* The infections are described by location.

Tinea corporis can involve any part of the body. The lesions are oval to round, red, and scaling patches with a central area of clearing (Fig. 23–1). The patterns can be polycyclic. **Tinea cruris**, or jock itch, appears as diffuse redness and scaling with sharp borders. **Tinea pedis**, or athlete's foot, appears in three forms. The most common, "moccasin foot," presents as scaling on the soles, sometimes with erythema and crusting. Intertriginous infection manifests as fissuring and scaling between the toes—usually the fourth and fifth toes. Inflammatory and vesicular infection occurs on the instep and sole. Moccasin foot often appears along with **tinea manuum**, in which the "two-feet–one-hand" pattern is common and is a clue to diagnosis (Fig. 23–2).

Tinea capitis is generally limited to children. Tinea tonsurans causes the so-called black dot type of tinea capitis, in which broken hairs appear as dark spots on the scalp. When the infection is caused by *Microsporon canis*, there are scaling and well-defined patches of hair loss with broken hairs. With more inflammation and infection, a red boggy area, a kerion, may develop.

Figure 23–1 Tinea corporis due to *Microsporon canis* showing red rings with peripheral scale and central clearing.

Figure 23–2   Dermatophyte infection with two-feet–one-hand pattern; right hand infected.

Figure 23–3   Hyphae diagnostic of dermatophyte infection (10% potassium hydroxide).

TABLE 23–1	Antifungal Creams	
Class	**Schedule**	**Brand**
Imidazole		
Clotrimazole 1%	Twice daily	Generic available
Econazole 1%	Once daily	Generic available[a]
Ketoconazole 2%	Once daily	Generic available
Miconazole 2%	Twice daily	Generic available
Oxiconazole 1%	Once daily	Oxistat
Allylamine		
Naftifine 1%	Once daily	Naftin
Terbinafine 1%	Twice daily	Lamisil

[a] Should be used twice daily for *Candida* infection.

DIFFERENTIAL DIAGNOSIS

Tinea corporis may be confused with contact dermatitis or atopic dermatitis, as can tinea cruris and tinea pedis. Jock itch can mimic intertrigo due to tight underwear. Tinea pedis can mimic psoriasis. Tinea capitis is sometimes confused with alopecia areata or seborrheic dermatitis. Tinea faciei is often mistaken for eczema.

HOW TO MAKE THE DIAGNOSIS

Clinical inspection is generally sufficient to make the diagnosis, but 10% potassium hydroxide scrapings showing branching hyphae or positive fungal cultures confirm the clinical impression (Fig. 23–3). The Wood's light examination for tinea capitis is only rarely helpful today because the causative agents are endothritic and do not fluoresce; however, *M. audouinii* and *M. canis* do fluoresce. An examination of plucked hairs and surrounding scalp scales often reveals organisms under the microscope.

TREATMENT

Fungal infections of the skin itself can be treated with topical antifungal creams of the imidazole or allylamine classes (Table 23–1). With more extensive or chronic involvement, oral agents such as Terbinafine 250 mg are taken daily for 3 to 4 weeks.

Tinea capitis requires oral griseofulvin (microsize), 10 to 15 mg/kg daily for at least 6 weeks, or terbinafine, 250 mg daily for 2 to 4 weeks. Absorption of griseofulvin increases if taken with fatty foods.

PROGNOSIS

Superficial fungal infections are readily cured with proper treatment.

Chapter 24

TINEA VERSICOLOR
(ICD-9 111.0)

Lawrence Charles Parish

SIGNS AND SYMPTOMS

Patients with tinea versicolor (TV) may complain of mild pruritus. Because the organism, *Malassezia furfur*, needs a warm, moist area high in lipids, TV often occurs in the warmer months or during the winter among patients who engage in vigorous exercise causing sweating. TV generally does not appear before puberty. It is characterized by sharply demarcated hyperpigmented or hypopigmented scaling patches on the trunk, neck, and proximal areas of the arms (Fig. 24–1). It is called "versicolor" because the coloring can be whitish, brownish, or even reddish, depending on the normal color of the patient's skin. The lesions give a fine, bran-like scale with minimal scratching. Patients are frequently not aware of the condition until they are suntanned and the hypopigmentation caused by TV becomes more noticeable.

DIFFERENTIAL DIAGNOSIS

Because the scaling is mild, TV can be confused with a drug eruption, neurodermatitis, or psoriasis, especially guttate psoriasis. If scaling is minimal, the hypopigmented patches may resemble vitiligo.

HOW TO MAKE THE DIAGNOSIS

An examination of the scales under the microscope using potassium hydroxide shows the characteristic hyphae and budding—"spaghetti and meatballs"—of TV (Fig. 24–2). The areas fluoresce green with a Wood's light.

Figure 24–1 Tinea versicolor. Sharply demarcated hyper- and hypopigmented patches on the trunk.

Figure 24-2 "Spaghetti and meatballs" of tinea versicolor (10% potassium hydroxide with Parker ink).

TREATMENT

There are many treatment regimens for TV. Antifungal creams of the imidazole or allylamines classes are all effective (Table 23–1). Remember that up to 10 g of cream is needed for each daily treatment. An older regimen is selenium sulfide shampoo, 2.5% daily for at least 2 weeks. A more efficient treatment is the oral administration of itraconazole 100 mg twice daily for 1 week.

PROGNOSIS

Scaling disappears in a few weeks, but pigmentation does not return to normal for several months. Unfortunately, although TV can be treated very effectively, it cannot be cured. Recurrences can occur annually for up to 20 years. Patients should be warned to expect recurrence in summer months or during the winter if they are devoted gym goers.

Chapter 25

SECONDARY SYPHILIS
(ICD-9 091.3)

John T. Crissey

SYMPTOMS AND SIGNS

The lesions of secondary syphilis (SS) are discrete asymptomatic, erythematous to copper-colored, macular, and maculopapular lesions, which present on the trunk and genitalia. A prodrome of sore throat and flu-like symptoms may precede the lesions by a few days. The face is usually heavily involved, especially in the seborrheic areas and along the hair line. Brownish or coppery macules and slightly scaly papules often appear on the palms and soles (Fig. 25–1). More than any other feature, these lesions should alert the examiner to the possibility of syphilis.

In other cases, SS lesions have a pronounced tendency to assume annular configurations, particularly in black patients. The face, anogenital areas, palms and soles, axillae, and periumbilical areas may be involved. Because of their size and configuration, these lesions are often called "nickel and dime syphilids" (Fig. 25–2). Mucous membrane lesions include a transient diffuse redness of the throat and the so-called mucous patches. The latter are slightly elevated round or oval papules, 5 to 12 mm in diameter, faintly inflammatory and covered with a pearly or grayish membrane. Lesions at the labial commissures may take the form of "split" or fissured papules, easily confused with ordinary perlèche. Mucocutaneous lesions in the genitalia and anal areas may appear as condylomata lata, which vary in morphology from slightly pedunculated, flat papules to smooth and button-like lesions or large cauliflower-like vegetations.

Figure 25–1 Secondary syphilis. Copper-colored macular lesions on palms and soles.

Figure 25-2 Secondary syphilis. Nickel and dime syphilid commonly presents on the face.

Other signs include more or less generalized nontender, rubbery lymphadenopathy, which occurs in approximately 85% of cases, and a nonscarring patchy or "moth-eaten" scalp alopecia.

Syphilis in patients infected with human immunodeficiency virus (HIV) presents special problems. Atypical clinical presentations are common, particularly ulcerating secondary lesions and pronounced systemic symptoms—the so-called malignant syphilis. Central nervous system (CNS) involvement is unusually common—16% to 40% in some studies.

DIFFERENTIAL DIAGNOSIS

Guttate psoriasis, pityriasis rosea, and widespread lichen planus sometimes resemble SS. The absence of other signs of SS help to establish the proper diagnosis.

HOW TO MAKE THE DIAGNOSIS

Syphilis is a laboratory diagnosis. The standard nontreponemal serologic test, the rapid plasma reagin (RPR), is positive in almost all cases of SS. To rule out false-positive reactions, a positive RPR should be confirmed by a treponemal test such as the microhemagglutination assay for *Treponema pallidum* (MHA-TP) before instituting treatment.

TREATMENT

SS can be treated successfully with intramuscular benzathine penicillin G, 2.4 million units once weekly for 2 weeks. Penicillin-allergic patients may be treated with oral tetracycline, 500 mg four times daily for 15 days. After treatment, titered RPR should be performed every 3 to 6 months for 2 years to rule out relapse or reinfection. In the presence of HIV infection, nontreponemal serologic tests are unreliable guides to treatment response, and conventional treatment schedules appear to be inadequate. Current literature should be consulted for the latest in the proper management of these difficult cases.

PROGNOSIS

The response to the treatment in otherwise healthy patients is excellent. Prognosis in patients with acquired immunodeficiency syndrome (AIDS) is guarded.

Section III

Blisters

Chapter 26

BULLOUS PEMPHIGOID
(ICD-9 694.4)

Jeffrey P. Callen

SYMPTOMS AND SIGNS

Bullous pemphigoid (BP) is often pruritic. Patients are usually over 60 years of age and present with tense bullae on normal skin (Fig. 26–1) or on an urticarial lesion. The bullae are subepidermal and eventually break, leaving an erosion. Healing occurs with temporary dyspigmentation, but without scarring. Mucous membranes are rarely affected in BP. However, a variant known as *benign mucous membrane pemphigoid* (cicatricial pemphigoid) affects the mucosal surfaces primarily, the mouth and eyes most often, and can result in blindness. BP may be caused by thiazide diuretics, spironolactone, furosemide, captopril, penicillamine, phenothiazines, tricyclic antidepressants, or benzodiazepines. BP is not a marker for internal malignancy as previously believed.

DIFFERENTIAL DIAGNOSIS

Bullous impetigo may look like BP, although it is primarily in intertriginous areas and impetigo bullae are flaccid. Other rare, subepidermal blistering

Figure 26–1 Bullous pemphigoid. Tense bullae on normal-appearing skin.

disorders must be considered because therapy often differs. These include linear immunoglobulin A (IgA) bullous dermatosis, dermatitis herpetiformis, anti–epiligrin cicatricial pemphigoid, and epidermolysis bullosa acquisita. In patients without blisters, the differential diagnosis includes urticaria and insect bite reactions.

HOW TO MAKE THE DIAGNOSIS

Punch biopsies should include both an intact blister for routine processing and a biopsy of adjacent normal-appearing skin for immunofluorescence microscopy. Immunoflourescence testing is sent in Michel's transport media to a specialized laboratory. BP is characterized by the deposition of IgG in the lamina lucida part of the basement membrane. Serum for indirect immunofluorescence, looking for circulating anti–basement membrane antibodies, should also be sent to a specialized laboratory. Results of serum tests vary from one laboratory to the next. Therefore, the selection of an appropriate consultant is critical. Results that do not fit with the clinical diagnosis should be repeated.

TREATMENT

Patients with BP vary in symptomatology. This factor as well as their age and preexisting medical conditions should be considered when making a decision about therapy. Drugs that cause BP should be discontinued. Oral corticosteroids such as prednisone, 1 to 2 mg/kg daily, are almost always effective. However, in this population steroids frequently result in toxicity. In hospitalized patients the daily application of super-potent topical corticosteroids is useful and may be steroid-sparing, but this approach is rarely practical in the United States. Oral niacinamide, 500 mg three times daily, plus tetracycline, 500 mg three times daily, is sometimes a worthy alternative. Many patients are given immunosuppressive or cytotoxic agents for their steroid-sparing effect. Methotrexate, azathioprine, mycophenolate mofetil, and cyclosporine are among the favored choices.

PROGNOSIS

BP rarely threatens life. Control results in less risk of secondary infection that may complicate eroded skin. Often, the disease burns out in 3 to 5 years.

Chapter 27

IMPETIGO
(ICD-9 684)

James C. Shaw

SYMPTOMS AND SIGNS

Impetigo is a common superficial bacterial infection caused by either strepto-cocci or staphylococci, or both. Impetigo is usually symptomatic with itching and burning. It begins as one or more red papules and over 2 to 3 days expands to a crusted patch. The condition can be nonbullous or bullous. In nonbul-lous impetigo, there are circular patches of scaling, superficial erosions, and honey-colored crusts (Fig. 27–1). The patches are usually periorificial on the face, especially around the nose and mouth. Bullous impetigo presents as flaccid, pus-filled lakes, which are often eroded at the time of presentation. This form occurs most commonly in intertriginous areas (Fig. 27–2). Bullae are 1 to 3 cm in diameter. There are no constitutional symptoms. Children are affected most often.

DIFFERENTIAL DIAGNOSIS

Tinea faciale has a similar appearance on the face but is usually more pruritic, is not typically periorificial, and has less surface crust. Tinea faciale can be anywhere on the face. Herpes zoster vesicles are unilateral or dermatomal. Herpes simplex must also be considered, and herpes infection can develop secondary impetigo.

HOW TO MAKE THE DIAGNOSIS

Examination is usually sufficient to make the diagnosis of impetigo. The typical 2- to 3-day onset also helps make the diagnosis. A bacterial culture for group A β-hemolytic streptococci or *Staphylococcus aureus* can be obtained to

Figure 27–1 Nonbullous impetigo with scaling, superficial erosions, and honey-colored crusts.

Figure 27–2 Bullous impetigo with flaccid, pus-filled bullae, and eroded areas.

confirm the diagnosis. The specimen should be taken from the base of the lesion. Treatment should be started while awaiting culture results.

TREATMENT

The mainstay of treatment for impetigo is systemic antibiotics that cover both the streptococci and the staphylococci involved. Good choices for adults are dicloxacillin or cephalexin, 250 mg four times daily by mouth. For penicillin-allergic patients, oral erythromycin, 250 mg four times daily, can be used. Dosages for children must be calculated by body weight. Mupirocin ointment 2% four times daily has been used successfully as a single-drug therapy in mild cases. It can be initiated while awaiting culture results and sensitivities.

PROGNOSIS

Impetigo is highly contagious until therapy is started. Complete recovery is the norm and requires up to 2 weeks of treatment. Scarring is rare. Glomerulonephritis is an unusual complication of impetigo after infection with certain strains of *Streptococcus*.

Chapter 28

HERPES SIMPLEX
(ICD-9 054.9)

James C. Shaw

SYMPTOMS AND SIGNS

Primary herpes simplex virus (HSV) infection can be severe, with patients complaining of burning and pain in involved areas, malaise, or low-grade fever. One or 2 days later, lesions appear. Recurrent HSV causes tingling, burning, or itching 1 day before the lesions appear. HSV can cause chronic erosions in patients who are immunosuppressed.

HSV type 1 (HSV-1) commonly infects nongenital skin, usually the face and most often the lips or mouth. Oral HSV presents as multiple shallow ulcerations in the mouth or grouped clear vesicles on the vermilion border of the lip. Impetiginization is common (Fig. 28–1).

HSV type 2 (HSV-2) usually infects anogenital skin. It appears as grouped vesicles or papules, 1 to 4 mm in diameter on a red base (Fig. 28–2). Usually, there are five to ten lesions in the group. There may be considerable edema. Most individuals with HSV-2 do not present with a primary infection, but with a "first recurrence."

HSV may also infect by inoculation, causing herpetic whitlow on the fingers. This condition is seen most often in health care workers, particularly dentists, dental technicians, and anesthesiologists.

DIFFERENTIAL DIAGNOSIS

Patients with tinea faciale complain of more pruritus than patients with HSV and have deeper papules and erythema, and no vesicles. Impetigo has honey-colored crusts and pus. Herpes zoster lesions appear in many clusters following a dermatome. Aphthous ulcers are usually singular.

HOW TO MAKE THE DIAGNOSIS

HSV is often diagnosed clinically. Confirmation is through Tzanck preparation (microscopy) or direct fluorescent antibody from vesicle fluid or debris. A

Figure 28–1   HSV-1 most commonly affects the face and mouth.

Figure 28-2   HSV-2. Clear vesicles with superficial erosions on the penis.

Tzanck test can be completed within 30 minutes or less; direct fluorescent antibody (DFA), which is sent to a laboratory, usually requires 2 hours, and viral culture takes 1 to 3 days. To perform a Tzanck smear, unroof a vesicle and gently smear the scrapings from the base onto a glass microscope slide. Let dry and fix the specimen with absolute alcohol or gentle heat. Then, stain with any blue stain (5% methylene blue, Wright's, Giemsa's) for a few seconds, rinse, dry, and through immersion oil or oil and cover slip, look

Figure 28-3   Tzanck preparation reveals multinucleated, giant keratinocytes in both herpes simplex and herpes zoster infections (methylene blue).

for multinucleated keratinocytes which are pathognomonic for herpesvirus infection (Fig. 28–3).

TREATMENT

Treat early with oral agents to stop viral replication. After several days, the cellular damage has occurred and antiviral therapy may not help. For acute HSV, whether primary or recurrent, use oral acyclovir, 200 mg five times daily for 5 days, or valacyclovir, 1,000 mg twice daily for 5 days. Oral famciclovir, 125 mg twice daily for 5 days, may also be used for acute disease. For chronic suppressive therapy, acyclovir, 400 mg two or three times daily, or famciclovir 250 mg two times daily are effective.

PROGNOSIS

Because HSV is contagious, patients should avoid close contact with others during the acute phase until lesions are completely healed. Genital herpes infection in pregnant women can infect the baby perinatally, and patients should alert their obstetrician if they have any symptoms or signs of active genital HSV infection.

Chapter 29

HERPES ZOSTER
(ICD-9 053.9)

James C. Shaw

SYMPTOMS AND SIGNS

Herpes zoster (shingles) usually begins with a 1- to 2-day prodrome of pain or burning in a dermatomal distribution. The discomfort of zoster is deep like a neuralgia or superficial on the skin. The pain can be severe. In the chest or abdominal locations, prodromal pain can mimic cardiac, musculoskeletal, or intraperitoneal diseases.

The eruption consists of red papules or clear vesicles on a red base. The lesions, 2 to 4 mm in diameter, are frequently umbilicated, can be individual or grouped and are in a dermatomal distribution (Fig. 29–1). They often progress to confluent vesicles, which then erode and crust over. Secondary bacterial infection is common. Older patients are more likely to develop extensive involvement and severe pain. In severe cases and in immunocompromised patients, more than a single dermatome can be affected.

Herpes zoster is caused by the reactivation of varicella-zoster infection (chickenpox), usually suffered years before.

DIFFERENTIAL DIAGNOSIS

Herpes simplex recurrences are dermatomal, but typically appear on the lip or genitals. Insect bites, folliculitis, and tinea capitis can look the same as herpes zoster on the scalp. Cellulitis and erysipelas have considerable edema and erythema, especially when they affect the face. Human immunodeficiency virus (HIV) infection should be considered in all patients with herpes zoster.

HOW TO MAKE THE DIAGNOSIS

Herpes zoster is often a clinical diagnosis but can be confirmed by some laboratory tests. **Tzanck smear** confirms infection with herpesviruses but

Figure 29–1   Herpes zoster. Typical dermatomal distribution on the trunk.

cannot differentiate between herpes simplex virus (HSV) and varicella-zoster virus (VZV). Tzanck smear is performed by unroofing a vesicle, scraping the base and smearing onto a glass slide, fixing with gentle heat or air dry, and staining with 5% methylene blue or Giemsa to look for multinucleated keratinocytes (see Chapter 28). **Direct fluorescent antibody** test confirms the presence of VZV or HSV within several hours. The test is done by the laboratory on a smear obtained in the same manner as for the Tzanck test (Fig. 28–3), or from centrifuged viral culture fluid. Biopsies and cultures may confirm the diagnosis but require several days.

TREATMENT

Because herpes zoster is self-limited, treatment is based on severity. Early treatment reduces the incidence and degree of postherpetic neuralgia. The dose of oral acyclovir for immunocompetent patients is 800 mg five times daily for 5 to 7 days. An alternative is valacyclovir, 1,000 mg three times daily for 10 days, or famciclovir, 500 mg or 750 mg three times daily for 7 days. For immunosuppressed patients, acyclovir 500 mg/m^2 body surface area is given intravenously every 8 hours for 10 days.

For immunocompetent patients, adjunct systemic corticosteroids may reduce lesion healing time, acute neuritis, and the need for narcotic analgesia. One regimen is oral prednisone, 60 mg daily for 1 week followed by 30 mg daily for a second week together with antiviral agents.

Postherpetic neuralgia may require treatment with narcotic analgesics or tricyclic antidepressants such as amitriptyline 50 mg to 100 mg daily by mouth.

Oral antibacterial antibiotics are needed only if there is evidence of secondary infection: dicloxacillin, cephalexin, or erythromycin, 250 mg four times daily are equally effective.

PROGNOSIS

Most cases of herpes zoster resolve with only mild scarring. Involvement of the tip of the nose is an important sign of potential corneal or conjunctival involvement because of the involvement of the ophthalmic branch of the trigeminal nerve, and ophthalmologic consultation is warranted. Ramsay Hunt syndrome (partial facial palsy) may occur when there is involvement of the geniculate ganglion. Recurrences are uncommon because immunity is boosted by an episode of herpes zoster. Postherpetic neuralgia is common in geriatric patients with severe disease. Immunocompromised patients can experience severe local or disseminated disease.

Herpes zoster is contagious to those who have not had varicella. Transmission is by direct contact with lesions.

Chapter 30

PEMPHIGUS VULGARIS
(ICD-9 694.5)

Jeffrey P. Callen

SYMPTOMS AND SIGNS

Pemphigus is a blistering disease of the skin and mucous membranes. There are at least two major variants: pemphigus vulgaris (PV) and pemphigus foliaceus (PF). Most patients are between the ages of 40 and 60. Patients with PV often present with painful oral ulcers (Fig. 30–1). The mouth sores or desquamative gingivitis are followed by skin lesions including flaccid bullae, which may be so fragile that they are sometimes not observed, and only erosions and crusts are seen (Fig. 30–2). Oral PV can develop by itself in the absence of skin disease. In contrast, the lesions of PF are superficial, are localized to the head, neck, and upper trunk, and rarely involve the mouth.

DIFFERENTIAL DIAGNOSIS

Impetigo and impetiginized eczema have typical honey-colored crusts. Seborrheic dermatitis is scaling. Bullous pemphigoid lesions are tense and not flaccid, and oral disease is rare. Aphthous stomatitis lesions are punched out. Patients with erosive oral lichen planus usually have typical violaceous papules on the skin. Oral erythema multiforme is often accompanied by skin erythema or target lesions. Herpes simplex virus infection tends to occur on the vermilion border of the lower lip and usually manifests in younger individuals. Paraneoplastic pemphigus (PNP) is a recently described entity that might mimic PV, lichen planus, or erythema multiforme. PNP is associated with a history of or an existing lymphoma or Castleman's disease.

Figure 30–1 Pemphigus vulgaris. Painful ulcerations in the mouth.

Figure 30-2   Pemphigus vulgaris. Severe erosions and crusts in the axilla.

HOW TO MAKE THE DIAGNOSIS

Punch biopsy of the skin or oral lesions demonstrates the intraepidermal blister. An additional biopsy for immunofluorescence microscopy of adjacent normal skin or mucosa (sent in Michel's transport media to a special laboratory) demonstrates the intraepidermal deposition of immunoglobulin, usually immunoglobulin G (IgG). Indirect immunofluorescence of the serum measures circulating antibodies and an enzyme-linked immunosorbent assay (ELISA) for desmoglein 3 titers correlates with the disease activity.

TREATMENT

Systemic corticosteroids, such as prednisone, 1 to 2 mg/kg daily, is usually required for PV. Patients with PF may respond to lower doses of oral corticosteroids. Corticosteroid-sparing regimens for either PV or PF include oral niacinamide, 500 mg three times daily, plus tetracycline, 500 mg three times daily, or intramuscular gold, 50 mg weekly and are effective in some patients. More reliable results occur with immunosuppressive and cytotoxic agents such as azathioprine, mycophenolate mofetil, methotrexate, chlorambucil, or cyclophosphamide. Rituximab therapy has been recently reported to be helpful in controlling pemphigus. Lastly, intravenous immune globulin therapy has been useful in some patients. Treatment is continued until clinical remission accompanied by negative indirect immunofluorescence testing for desmoglein 3 antibodies.

PROGNOSIS

Untreated PV can be fatal when complicated by infection or fluid imbalance. PF has a better prognosis, and patients rarely die from it. In both PV and PF, it is possible for spontaneous resolution to occur in some patients after 3 to 5 years.

Chapter 31

TOXIC EPIDERMAL NECROLYSIS/STEVENS–JOHNSON SYNDROME
(ICD-9 695.1)

Jeffrey P. Callen

SYMPTOMS AND SIGNS

Toxic epidermal necrolysis (TEN) and Stevens–Johnson syndrome (SJS) are two terms that describe the clinical spectrum of a severe, life-threatening, blistering disorder of the skin and mucous membranes. Historically, more extensive skin loss (greater than 30% of body surface) is labeled TEN, whereas SJS is usually associated with less than 10% of body surface skin loss (see Chapter 16). In TEN/SJS, there is often a 1- to 3-day prodrome period of fever, conjunctivitis, pharyngitis, or pruritus. Frank skin pain and tenderness constitute an ominous sign. Mucosal surfaces of the mouth, eyes, genitalia, and anus are affected early in the disease (Fig. 31–1). Shortly thereafter, the patient develops widespread bullae that are easily ruptured; target lesions may also be seen (Fig. 31–2). The bullae can be extended laterally when pressed down upon, or the skin may tear when it is rubbed (Nikolsky's sign). TEN/SJS may progress dramatically to sheets of skin loss (Fig. 31–3).

Fluid and electrolyte balance, poor thermoregulation, and bacterial infections may result from the skin loss. Skin healing occurs with dyspigmentation but minimal, if any, scarring. Ocular involvement can result in blindness.

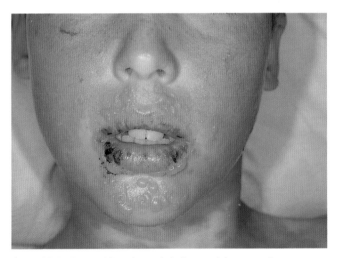

Figure 31–1 Toxic epidermal necrolysis/Stevens–Johnson syndrome (TEN/SJS). Mucosal blisters and erythematous patches on the skin.

Figure 31–2 Toxic epidermal necrolysis/Stevens–Johnson syndrome (TEN/SJS). Target lesions and bullae on the hands and arms of the patient in Figure 31–1.

Figure 31–3 Toxic epidermal necrolysis/Stevens–Johnson syndrome (TEN/SJS). Skin is lost in sheets in severe cases.

TEN and SJS are rare disorders and almost always are a manifestation of an adverse drug reaction. The most common offending drugs are antibiotics (sulfonamides, penicillins, cephalosporins), anticonvulsants (phenytoin, phenobarbital, carbamazepine), nonsteroidal anti-inflammatory agents, and allopurinol. Many other drugs have been implicated, including systemic corticosteroids. TEN/SJS occurs more commonly in human immunodeficiency virus (HIV)-infected individuals or in those on any immunosuppressive or cytotoxic therapy.

DIFFERENTIAL DIAGNOSIS

TEN and SJS are distinctive and dramatic once they are manifest fully. Early in their evolution, they may be confused with erythema multiforme, paraneoplastic pemphigus, or a morbilliform drug eruption. Other blistering diseases, specifically drug-induced linear immunoglobulin A (IgA) bullous dermatosis, must also be considered, particularly if there is an atypical presentation. Staphylococcal scalded skin syndrome, which occurs most often in children, is more superficial and can be distinguished on skin biopsy.

HOW TO MAKE THE DIAGNOSIS

Punch biopsy can help confirm the clinical diagnosis of TEN/SJS. Immunofluorescence microscopy will aid in the distinction from other blistering diseases.

TREATMENT

TEN and SJS are usually drug-related, and suspect drugs should be stopped. Patients should be admitted to a burn unit or an intensive care unit with experience in caring for such patients. Careful attention to infection and fluid and electrolyte balance are necessary. Many approaches to dressing and cleansing have been championed in the literature. However, none has been tested in a scientific manner or adequately compared. Ophthalmologic examination and early intervention may prevent scarring and blindness.

Drug treatment is controversial. Most authorities in the United States consider corticosteroids to be contraindicated, and if they are to be useful, then they must be given in high doses; methylprednisone, 2 mg/kg per day intravenously the first 24 to 48 hours. Cytotoxic or immunosuppressive therapies are unproven. Plasmapheresis has also been suggested as part of early management. Intravenous immunoglobulin (IVIg), 0.75 g/kg per day for 4 to 5 days, has recently been demonstrated to result in rapid control and speedy healing in most studies conducted in the United States; however studies from Europe suggest that patients treated with IVIg fare less well than those treated with corticosteroids.

PROGNOSIS

Mortality is 30% overall, but higher in elderly patients with multiple preexisting medical conditions. In patients who do survive there is a high rate of ocular complications, even when aggressive therapies have been utilized.

Chapter 32

SEBORRHEIC KERATOSIS
(ICD-9 702.19)

James C. Shaw

SYMPTOMS AND SIGNS

Seborrheic keratoses are common benign skin growths. Mostly asymptomatic and only occasionally pruritic, they can manifest as solitary or multiple lesions. Common sites include the head, neck, and back. They are usually verrucous, scaling, and sharply differentiated from the surrounding skin (Fig. 32–1). The color varies from flesh-colored to black or even red, if irritated or inflamed. Seborrheic keratoses can be flat or raised and range in size from less than 0.5 cm to more than 3 cm in diameter. Slow enlargement over the years is normal. Rapid development of multiple lesions occurs rarely (Leser–Trélat sign) and can be a paraneoplastic phenomenon associated with gastric and

Figure 32–1   Seborrheic keratosis. Verrucous, scaling, light brown, "stuck-on" lesion.

other adenocarcinomas. A variant, called **dermatosis papulosa nigra**, appears as multiple small, dark seborrheic keratoses on the faces of African Americans. Stucco keratoses are multiple, white 0.2- to 0.4-cm seborrheic keratoses on the lower legs or arms. The cause of seborrheic keratoses is unknown but there has been recent evidence suggesting a possible contributing role for some strains of wart virus.

DIFFERENTIAL DIAGNOSIS

Common warts have a more papillomatous surface with many black dots visible on their surface. These are thrombosed vessels. Squamous cell carcinoma *in situ* **(Bowen's disease)** is a reddish brown patch of hyperkeratosis, often on sun-exposed skin. Rarely, a black seborrheic keratosis can resemble malignant melanoma.

HOW TO MAKE THE DIAGNOSIS

Diagnosis of seborrheic keratosis is clinical. Excisional biopsy is necessary if malignant melanoma is suspected.

TREATMENT

Treatment for seborrheic keratosis is generally not required and tends to be for cosmetic purposes. Methods include cryotherapy, electrodesiccation, and curettage, or shave excision.

PROGNOSIS

Untreated lesions persist and may enlarge slowly over the years. Large lesions can become traumatized, pruritic, or rarely secondarily infected. There appears to be no risk of malignant degeneration beyond that of normal skin.

Chapter 33

SQUAMOUS CELL CARCINOMA
(ICD-9 173.3 FACE; 173.4 SCALP, NECK; 173.5 TRUNK; 173.6 UPPER EXTREMITY; 173.7 LOWER EXTREMITY)

David H. Frankel

SYMPTOMS AND SIGNS

Squamous cell carcinoma (SCC) of the skin is often asymptomatic, although patients may complain of itching or pain. SCC appears as a scaling, hyperkeratotic papule or nodule (Fig. 33–1). It is usually on sun-exposed skin and may ulcerate. Occasionally, SCC develops in sites of chronic inflammation or ulceration, as in discoid lupus erythematosus or hidradenitis suppurativa, or in sites of radiation therapy or burn. In these instances, the clinical appearance may be more subtle. Such SCCs are at high risk for recurrence or metastasis. Other high-risk sites are the lower lip, ear, digits, scalp, and penis. Recurrent SCC must also be considered in the high-risk group.

DIFFERENTIAL DIAGNOSIS

Keratoacanthoma may be undistinguishable from SCC, unless it has the characteristic central keratin plug. Biopsy is often necessary to distinguish between the two. Seborrheic keratoses appear greasy, "stuck on," and warty. Verrucae are also scaling but, when shaved, reveal the telltale black dots of thrombosed blood vessels.

HOW TO MAKE THE DIAGNOSIS

Punch biopsy or shave biopsy is needed to confirm the diagnosis of SCC.

Figure 33–1 Squamous cell carcinoma. High-risk lesion on the lip.

TREATMENT

Data on cure rates of various therapies for SCC are difficult to summarize because the number of variables and risk factors is great. Cure rates for all modalities are nearly 90% when the modality suits the type of SCC being treated. Cryotherapy or electrodesiccation and curettage should be used only for superficial, small, low-risk lesions. Surgical excision and primary closure, the time-honored method, is more likely to be curative for higher-risk lesions and has the advantage that excision margins can be evaluated by the pathologist. Remember that excised lesions with positive margins must be re-excised until the margins are negative. Mohs' micrographic surgery is reserved for high-risk lesions, in which the cure rate—even for difficult tumors—can be as high as 95%. Radiation therapy is generally reserved for large lesions in the elderly.

PROGNOSIS

The risk of local recurrence after treatment is greatest for SCC in high-risk sites or in SCCs that are large (over 1 cm in diameter), poorly differentiated, or invasive to the deep dermis or fat, or that have invaded the perineurium. Overall, the 5-year rate of metastasis is approximately 5% for SCC on sun-damaged skin. Rates are higher for high-risk tumors. Approximately one third of patients with SCC develop another SCC within 5 years. Affected patients should have yearly follow-up to check for recurrence, new tumors, or lymph node metastasis.

Chapter 34

ACTINIC KERATOSIS
(ICD-9 702.2)

David H. Frankel

SYMPTOMS AND SIGNS

Actinic keratoses (AK), in general, are asymptomatic. Sometimes patients complain of itching or burning but when present, these symptoms should be considered signs of possible transformation to squamous cell carcinoma (SCC). AK present as small, 3- to 6-mm, red, rough, poorly circumscribed patches on sun-exposed skin (Fig. 34–1). Common sites include the nose, tips of the ears, forehead, forearms, and hands. AK are extremely common in the elderly, although given the population growth in the US sunbelt, it is not uncommon to see them in young adults. Most AK do not progress to SCC and, with scrupulous sun protection, some small and superficial lesions will resolve spontaneously. Lesions that grow rapidly, ulcerate, thicken, or become symptomatic should be held in suspicion as possible early SCCs.

The equivalent of AK on the lip, actinic cheilitis, is a premalignant condition characterized by loss of the vermilion border, milky discoloration, and scaling. **It is seen** most often on the lower lip.

DIFFERENTIAL DIAGNOSIS

Occasionally, small patches of eczema or psoriasis may look like AK. In general, however, eczema is more pruritic than AK and psoriasis is unlikely

Figure 34–1 Actinic keratoses. Multiple, red, scaling, poorly circumscribed lesions on sun-exposed skin.

to be limited to sun-exposed areas, especially because sunlight ameliorates psoriasis. Bowen's disease, or SCC *in situ* may have a very similar appearance to AK or to seborrheic keratosis, but it is often larger that a few millimeters.

HOW TO MAKE THE DIAGNOSIS

Finding typical lesions on sun-exposed skin is enough to make the diagnosis of AK. Punch or shave biopsy is recommended when either SCC or Bowen's disease are suspected.

TREATMENT

AK that persist beyond 1 month should be treated with light cryotherapy or light electrodesiccation and curettage. Fluorouracil solution 2% or 5%, or cream 5%, applied twice daily for up to 3 weeks may be used for patients with numerous lesions. Patients should be warned that fluorouracil often causes contact dermatitis and photosensitivity. Actinic cheilitis can be treated similarly to AK, but laser or surgical vermilionectomy is sometimes necessary to eradicate severe disease.

PROGNOSIS

Patients with AK respond well to therapy. However, they are likely to develop new lesions, and yearly follow-up is reasonable.

Chapter 35

KERATOACANTHOMA
(ICD-9 238.2)

James C. Shaw

SYMPTOMS AND SIGNS

Keratoacanthomas (KA) are usually asymptomatic and develop rapidly over 2 to 6 weeks. The rapid enlargement of a dome-shaped nodule of up to 1 cm in diameter with a central keratin-filled plug is typical (Fig. 35–1). KA usually appear on sun-exposed areas of the face, neck, arms, and hands. Rare syndromes exist in which multiple KA develop. The Ferguson–Smith type of KA consists of multiple, large KA; the Gryzbowski type consists of multiple, eruptive small lesions.

DIFFERENTIAL DIAGNOSIS

Squamous cell carcinoma (SCC) can appear identical to KA, but the growth of SCC is usually slower. Molluscum contagiosum can resemble small KA, but molluscum lesions usually remain small—2 to 3 mm in diameter.

Figure 35–1 Keratoacanthoma. Rapidly developing, dome-shaped papule or nodule with central keratin plug on sun-damaged skin.

HOW TO MAKE THE DIAGNOSIS

Diagnosis of KA is usually made by history and examination. However, if SCC is a possibility, a shave or excisional biopsy must be done to confirm the diagnosis.

TREATMENT

KA may resolve spontaneously, leaving depressed, atrophic scars. However, because of the clinical and histologic similarity to SCC, plus rare reports of metastases, most authors consider KA to be a variant of SCC and therefore treat KA with ablative therapies. The treatment of choice is excision. Alternatives include intralesional methotrexate, 5-fluorouracil, or interferon-α-2a, systemic retinoids (especially for multiple KA), or radiation therapy.

PROGNOSIS

Complete excision is usually curative. Recurrences can develop at the site of treated lesions.

Chapter 36

BASAL CELL CARCINOMA
(ICD-9 173.3 HEAD, EAR; 173.4 SCALP, NECK; 173.5 TRUNK; 173.6 UPPER EXTREMITY; 173.7 LOWER EXTREMITY)

James C. Shaw

SYMPTOMS AND SIGNS

The presentation of basal cell carcinoma (BCC), the most common human cancer, is an asymptomatic papule that often goes unnoticed by patients. The typical presentation is an enlarging papule or a sore that does not heal and bleeds easily—the so-called rodent ulcer (Fig. 36–1). The sun-exposed areas of the head and neck are the most common sites involved. A papule or plaque with a pearly or translucent appearance and crossed by telangiectasias is highly suggestive. Superficial BCCs resemble a patch of dermatitis with a pearly rim (Fig. 36–2). Sclerosing BCCs are insidious and hard to diagnose. They are white to yellow and often indistinguishable from common scar tissue (Fig. 36–3). Pigmented BCCs resemble nodular malignant melanoma (Fig. 36–4). Patients who received therapeutic radiation (in the 1950s and 1960s) for acne or tinea capitis are at high risk for the development of multiple BCCs.

Figure 36–1 Basal cell carcinoma. "Rodent ulcer" (left nostril) next to typical pearly papule with telangiectasias.

Figure 36–2 Superficial basal cell carcinoma resembles dermatitis, but with raised, pearly border.

Figure 36–3 Sclerosing basal cell carcinoma can be mistaken for scar tissue.

Figure 36–4 Pigmented basal cell carcinoma resembles nodular malignant melanoma.

DIFFERENTIAL DIAGNOSIS

Flesh-colored nevi can resemble BCCs, as can other benign lesions such as neurofibromas, hidrocystomas, and lichen planus–like keratoses. Hyperkeratotic BCCs can be confused with squamous cell carcinoma.

HOW TO MAKE THE DIAGNOSIS

Most BCCs can be identified by physical examination with magnification and good lighting. Dermatoscopy can help differentiate pigmented BCC from melanoma by demonstrating round pigment globules (see Chapter 39). Histologic confirmation by either shave or punch biopsy is indicated to confirm the diagnosis and assess histologic subtypes, which include nodular, sclerosing, and superficial types.

TREATMENT

Treatment options for BCC include surgical excision, Mohs' micrographic surgery, radiation therapy, and destructive modalities such as electrodesiccation and curettage or cryotherapy. Although there is literature to support all modalities, the best method is probably surgical excision, because this allows histologic confirmation of excision margins. Remember that excised lesions with positive margins must be re-excised. Mohs' micrographic surgery is indicated for high-risk lesions about the central face and ears, for sclerosing BCCs, for recurrent BCCs, and for BCCs with aggressive histologic features. Radiation therapy is reserved for elderly patients.

PROGNOSIS

The combined cure rate of primary BCCs is greater than 90% and greater than 95% with Mohs' surgery. For recurrent BCCs, Mohs' surgery has a 5-year cure rate of approximately 94%, compared with 90% for radiation, 83% for excision, and 60% for electrodesiccation and curettage. It is worthwhile to remember that nearly one third of patients with BCCs develop another BCC within 5 years. This is especially common in patients with a history of radiation therapy. BCCs rarely metastasize.

Chapter 37

MELANOCYTIC NEVUS
(ICD-9 216.3 FACE; 216.4 SCALP, NECK; 216.5 TRUNK; 216.6 UPPER EXTREMITY; 216.7 LOWER EXTREMITY)

David H. Frankel

SYMPTOMS AND SIGNS

Junctional, compound, and intradermal nevi are benign lesions and should not be symptomatic. Symptoms such as itching or pain may indicate transformation to malignant melanoma (MM). **Junctional nevi** are usually macules, although sometimes they are slightly elevated. **Compound nevi** are macules or papules. **Intradermal nevi** are papular. Both lesions are symmetric, have sharp borders, and are uniformly pigmented tan to dark brown or even black (Fig. 37–1). Intradermal nevi may be nonpigmented, pink, or tan (Fig. 37–2). They are also sharp-bordered, generally measure 1 to 6 mm in diameter, and do not undergo rapid enlargement or other sudden changes in appearance.

DIFFERENTIAL DIAGNOSIS

There are many benign pigmented lesions to consider in the differential diagnosis of melanocytic nevi, including dermatofibroma, lentigo, angioma, postinflammatory hyperpigmentation, skin tag, and others. Any

Figure 37–1 Melanocytic nevus. This compound nevus on the foot is symmetric, sharply bordered, uniformly pigmented, 3 mm in diameter, and without a history of rapid enlargement.

Figure 37–2   Melanocytic nevus. Intradermal nevus with no ABCDE changes.

lesions with "ABCDE" features must be biopsied to rule out MM (**ABCDE**: **A**symmetry, **B**order irregularity, **C**olor variegation, **D**iameter greater than 6 mm, **E**nlargement over a 1- or 2-month period; see Chapter 39). Most benign nevi appear before the age of 35 years. Pigmented lesions appearing in persons older than 35 should be suspected of being MM.

HOW TO MAKE THE DIAGNOSIS

If the lesion is asymptomatic and there are no ABCDE changes, the diagnosis can be made clinically. If MM is suspected, the diagnosis must be made by excisional biopsy.

TREATMENT

Benign nevi are removed for cosmetic reasons. This can be accomplished by shave, punch, or elliptical technique.

PROGNOSIS

Melanocytic nevi are benign lesions that may become MMs at any time. Patients should be taught the importance of self-examination and early signs of MM.

Chapter 38

HALO NEVUS
(ICD-9 M8723/0)

John T. Crissey

SIGNS AND SYMPTOMS

Itching and varying degrees of erythema may precede or accompany the development of the characteristic depigmented ring of the halo nevus (HN). The halo is several millimeters to centimeters wide and surrounds a preexisting pigmented nevus (Fig. 38–1). The halo usually reaches its maximum size in 1 or 2 months, after which the central nevus slowly diminishes in size and over a period of months or years tends to disappear. The depigmented area eventually resumes its normal color. The condition is common and usually occurs in children and young adults. The incidence of HN is high—nearly 25%—in patients with vitiligo, and HN may be a forerunner of that disease.

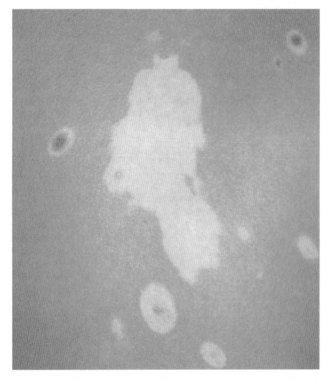

Figure 38–1 Halo nevus surrounded by zones of depigmentation; patient also has a large patch of vitiligo.

HN is a benign junctional, dermal, or compound nevocellular nevus undergoing morphologic and pathologic changes in response to an immunologic process not yet fully understood.

DIFFERENTIAL DIAGNOSIS

Zones of depigmentation can occur around malignant melanoma, blue nevus, dermatofibroma, and neurofibroma.

HOW TO MAKE THE DIAGNOSIS

When the clinical picture of HN is typical, the history and appearance should suffice. If the central nevus shows signs suggestive of malignant melanoma—asymmetry, irregular border, variations in color, diameter greater than 6 mm, or a history of sudden growth—an excisional biopsy is indicated.

TREATMENT

Typical cases need no treatment other than reassurance. Nevertheless, patients should be informed of the possibility of developing vitiligo and reexamined at 6-month intervals for 1 year to be certain that resolution is occurring.

PROGNOSIS

Repigmentation usually takes months to years.

Chapter 39

MALIGNANT MELANOMA
(ICD-9 172.3 Face; 172.4 Scalp, Neck; 172.5 Trunk; 172.6 Upper Extremity; 172.7 Lower Extremity)

James C. Shaw

SYMPTOMS AND SIGNS

Malignant melanoma (MM) is usually asymptomatic. Sometimes it can cause pruritus. Pruritus in a "mole" is a cardinal symptom that cannot be ignored. Bleeding is also an important complaint. MM usually develops as a patch, papule, or nodule. It is almost always pigmented, although nonpigmented **(amelanotic MM)** forms can arise. MM develops in preexisting nevi or *de novo* on normal skin. Current estimates are that 1 in 75 Americans will develop MM during their lifetime. The **ABCDE** of diagnosis are crucial to both physicians and patients (Figs. 39–1 through 39–4):

    Asymmetry

    Border irregularities

    Color variegation, including blue, gray, red, and black

    Diameter usually greater than 6 mm

    Enlargement, either of an existing nevus or of a new lesion, over a 1- or 2-month period

Figure 39–1 Malignant melanoma. **A**symmetry, **B**order irregularity, **C**olor variegation, **D**iameter, **E**nlargement (by history) of malignant melanoma.

Figure 39–2   ABCDE all present in this malignant melanoma.

Figure 39–3   Rapidly growing nodular malignant melanoma.

Figure 39–4 Melanoma, diascopy.

DIFFERENTIAL DIAGNOSIS

Darkly pigmented seborrheic keratoses, pigmented basal cell carcinomas (BCCs), and darkly pigmented atypical nevi commonly resemble MM. Pyogenic granulomas resemble amelanotic melanoma. Blue nevi, common in Asians, also look like MM.

Dermatoscopy utilizes optical enhancement called **epiluminescence microscopy** to identify features that help diagnose melanomas clinically and differentiate them from other pigmented lesions. With some training, characteristic morphologic features of MM versus benign nevi or pigmented BCC can be recognized (Fig. 39–4). Dermatoscopy can often help clinicians decide whether or not to biopsy a pigmented lesion.

HOW TO MAKE THE DIAGNOSIS

Histologic confirmation is essential for the diagnosis of MM. Biopsies must include epidermis, dermis, and subcutaneous fat. Excisional biopsy is preferable, but incisional biopsy is indicated in large lesions, especially when MM is suspected in large facial lesions. Shallow shave biopsies should not be done. A shave may not reach the base of the lesion; therefore, the precise millimeter of the depth of tumor invasion cannot be estimated. Knowledge of the depth of invasion is essential for proper staging and treatment (see Section "Prognosis"). Sentinel lymph node biopsy is increasingly used in patients with a proven melanoma greater than 1 mm deep. This method uses dye and isotope mapping to disclose the sentinel node.

TREATMENT

Surgical excision of primary cutaneous melanoma is the treatment of choice for MM. Current recommendations on margins are 0.5 cm for melanoma *in situ* (epidermal only), 1 cm for MM less than 1.5 mm deep, 1 to 2 cm for lesions 1.51 to 4 mm deep, and 2 to 3 cm for lesions deeper than 4 mm. Lymph node dissection is indicated when there is proven metastasis to a single drainage basin, and in some cases of intermediate depth (1.5 mm to 4 mm deep). High dose interferon-α is the only adjuvant therapy proven to be effective. Chemotherapy is used in metastatic disease and as palliative treatment.

Preventive measures are vital. Sun protection beginning in infancy may be the most effective measure. Sun-protective behavior includes avoidance of direct sun exposure, especially between 10 AM and 3 PM, and careful use of protective clothing, hats, and sun blocks. Skin self-examination for early detection is also important, especially for patients with numerous moles or with the atypical mole syndrome. Monthly total body examination with lighting and mirrors or with assistants often detect early lesions that can be cured.

PROGNOSIS

The depth of tumor invasion is the best predictor of long-term survival. Approximate 5-year survival figures are over 95% for tumors 0.75 mm deep, 85% for tumors 0.76 to 1.49 mm, 75% for tumors 1.50 to 2.49 mm, 65% for tumors 2.5 to 3.99, and 45% for tumors deeper than 4 mm. Five-year survival drops to 35% if there is nodal involvement and to 5% if there is distant metastasis. Younger patients and women may have more favorable outcomes. MM on the hands, feet, or mucosa have a worse prognosis.

Chapter 40

DYSPLASTIC NEVUS
(ICD-9 238.9)

James C. Shaw

SYMPTOMS AND SIGNS

Dysplastic nevi (DN), also called **Clark's nevi**, or atypical nevi, are asymptomatic. Patients may have only a single lesion or hundreds of them. DN are macules at least 5 mm in diameter with variable pigmentation, indistinct margins, and irregular, asymmetric outline (Fig. 40–1). Pigmentation frequently includes shades of brown and red and occasionally some black. The pigment variability is usually less than what is seen with malignant melanoma. The most common site is the back. Patients with many lesions (**dysplastic nevus syndrome**) have DN anywhere on the trunk and also on the proximal extremities and scalp (Fig. 40–2). Pruritus or bleeding in any nevus may be associated with transformation to melanoma.

DIFFERENTIAL DIAGNOSIS

Common melanocytic nevi are sometimes irregularly pigmented, but more typically tan to dark brown. They also have distinct margins, regular outlines, and raised contour and measure less than 5 mm in diameter. **Halo nevi** are surrounded by a white ring of depigmentation. Malignant melanomas have many of the features of dysplastic nevi, and may be impossible to differentiate from dysplastic nevi on clinical examination.

Figure 40–1   Dysplastic nevus with variegated pigmentation and irregular borders. Malignant melanoma was ruled out by excisional biopsy.

Figure 40–2 Patient with the dysplastic nevus syndrome presenting with many lesions on the trunk.

HOW TO MAKE THE DIAGNOSIS

Clinical features are often enough to make a diagnosis. Dermatoscopy can be helpful in differentiating DN from melanoma (see Chapter 39). However, punch or excisional biopsy of the entire lesion is mandatory for any lesion that appears suspicious for malignant melanoma. Destructive treatments such as cryotherapy, electrodesiccation, and carbon dioxide laser ablation are contraindicated because they will not provide histologic confirmation of the diagnosis.

TREATMENT

Patients should be taught the "**ABCDE**" (**A**symmetry, **B**order irregularity, **C**olor variegation, **D**iameter greater than 6 mm, **E**nlargement over a 1- or 2-month period) of malignant melanoma, the importance of sun protection, and the need to examine themselves every month. They should also be examined by their physician every 6 to 12 months. The use of selected or total body photography has been recommended in patients with large numbers of lesions.

Re-excision of DN with positive margins is controversial when there is significant malanocyte atypia. However, because the histologic diagnosis of DN is often made in the presence of only minimal atypia, close communication with the consulting dermatopathologist is essential to make sure DN are neither overtreated nor undertreated.

PROGNOSIS

Patients with multiple dysplastic nevi have an increased risk of developing melanoma. With a family history of melanoma as well, the relative risk is even greater. These patients must be carefully watched.

Chapter 41

DERMATOFIBROMA
(ICD-9 216.9)

James C. Shaw

SYMPTOMS AND SIGNS

Patients with dermatofibroma (DF) present with an asymptomatic smooth, firm, round, brownish papule or nodule, usually measuring less than 1 cm in diameter (Fig. 41–1). There is often a peripheral rim of hyperpigmentation. When DFs are pinched, they dimple in the center. DFs are most commonly found on the legs of women. They are thought to be fibrosing reactions to a local insult such as an arthropod bite or folliculitis.

DIFFERENTIAL DIAGNOSIS

Scars or keloids, if small and round, can mimic DF. They, however, do not dimple. Melanocytic nevi, melanomas, and solitary lesions of Kaposi's sarcoma can resemble a darkly pigmented dermatofibroma. In larger lesions, usually greater than 2 cm, dermatofibrosarcoma protuberans (DFSP) needs to be considered. DFSP is a locally aggressive malignant fibrosing neoplasm.

Figure 41–1 Dermatofibroma. Firm, brown papule with a peripheral rim of hyperpigmentation.

HOW TO MAKE THE DIAGNOSIS

Most DFs are detected by examination alone. The "dimple" is very helpful. A history of an unchanging lesion present for months to years supports the diagnosis. Punch or elliptical biopsy extending to subcutaneous fat is indicated if the diagnosis is in doubt.

TREATMENT

No treatment is necessary. In patients in whom the lesion causes symptoms such as pain or bleeding with leg shaving or if for cosmetic reasons it is unacceptable, the treatment is surgical excision and primary closure.

PROGNOSIS

DFs persist if not removed. Large numbers of DFs can be associated with systemic lupus erythematosus (SLE), and screening for SLE may be indicated in select patients.

Chapter 42

SKIN TAGS
(ICD-9 701.9)

Charles A. Gropper

SYMPTOMS AND SIGNS

Skin tags are asymptomatic. They are extremely common, small (1 to 3 mm), flesh-colored or brown papules. They are usually pedunculated (Fig. 42–1). Skin tags can occur anywhere on the body but are particularly common around the neck, in the groin or axillae, or under the breasts of women. They occur more often in people who are obese and tend to run in families.

DIFFERENTIAL DIAGNOSIS

Skin tags can be confused with seborrheic keratoses, neurofibromas, or nevi. Seborrheic keratoses often have a bumpy, **scaly** surface. Neurofibromas tend to be compressible and larger than skin tags. Nevi are frequently larger than skin tags and more darkly pigmented.

HOW TO MAKE THE DIAGNOSIS

The diagnosis is made on examination. It can be confirmed by shave biopsy.

Figure 42–1　Skin tag. Soft, flesh-colored, pedunculated papule.

TREATMENT

Skin tags are treated mainly for cosmetic reasons. Additional reasons for treating skin tags include color change, bleeding, itching, and interference with clothing. The lesions may be removed by shearing at the base with a scalpel or scissors. They can also be destroyed by light electrodesiccation or cryosurgery.

PROGNOSIS

Skin tags are benign lesions. Like any other skin growth or area of skin, they can rarely be the site of development of a malignancy, so the change of color should not be ignored. Any person who has a few skin tags will likely develop more as time progresses.

Chapter 43

EPIDERMOID CYST AND PILAR CYST
(ICD-9 706.2)

Charles A. Gropper

SYMPTOMS AND SIGNS

Cysts are asymptomatic until they become inflamed. They are among the most common skin lesions. Patients present with subcutaneous nodules that have the consistency of semifirm jelly, much like the feel of an eyeball. They are freely movable under the skin. Epidermoid cysts appear most commonly on the face, neck, upper trunk, and scrotum. They often have a visible central punctum (Fig. 43–1). Pilar cysts mainly occur on the scalp; multiple cysts are common. These cysts often lack a central punctum and are filled with keratin, which may have a slightly cheesy smell. Either type can rupture and become inflamed; frank infection with *Staphylococcus aureus* is less common. In either situation, the lesions become quite painful and drain serous or foul-smelling keratinaceous material.

Rarely, epidermoid cysts appear as a feature of syndromes. Gardner's syndrome consists of intestinal polyps, osteomas, fibromas, and epidermoid cysts. Basal cell nevus syndrome presents with multiple basal cell carcinomas, nevi, jaw cysts, and skeletal abnormalities.

Figure 43–1 Epidermoid cysts on the face. Note the central punctum on the upper lesion.

DIFFERENTIAL DIAGNOSIS

Furuncles can be easily confused with inflamed epidermoid cysts. Carcinomas of the lung, breast, and genitourinary system can metastasize to the scalp. These lesions, however, are firm and fixed.

HOW TO MAKE THE DIAGNOSIS

The diagnosis is suggested by the appearance and consistency of the lesion. The presence of a punctum is especially helpful. The diagnosis can be confirmed only by removal.

TREATMENT

Asymptomatic cysts need not be removed if they do not trouble the patient. It is helpful to remove cysts that become inflamed, but removal should be undertaken only after the inflammation has subsided for several weeks. Inflamed cysts often respond to high-dose oral erythromycin, 500 mg two to four times daily, because of its anti-inflammatory properties, and warm compresses. Alternatively, the lesions can be incised and drained or injected with a small amount (less than 0.5 mL) of intralesional triamcinolone acetonide solution in a concentration of 2.5 to 5.0 mg/mL. Infected cysts are treated in the same manner as furuncles.

PROGNOSIS

The prognosis of epidermoid cysts is variable. Some spontaneously regress, some persist without change, and some continue to grow. The particular course of any given lesion is not predictable. Although epidermoid cysts are always benign, there are extremely rare reports of cysts giving rise to squamous cell carcinoma.

Chapter 44

MOLLUSCUM CONTAGIOSUM
(ICD-9 078.0)

John T. Crissey

SYMPTOMS AND SIGNS

Molluscum contagiosum (MC) is an asymptomatic condition. Lesions are skin-colored, white, or slightly pink, flattened globose papules, 3 to 6 mm in diameter, many with a small central aperture or dell (Fig. 44–1). The surface is "semigloss," pearl-like, and waxy. Lesions may occur singly or in groups. Exposed surfaces are favored, but no area is exempt. The groin and genitalia are commonly involved in sexually active persons. Lesions undergoing spontaneous resolution often become acutely inflamed. Facial involvement in adults usually indicates concomitant human immunodeficiency virus (HIV) infection. Lesions in these cases may become very large and run together. MC is a viral infection, common in children and young adults, and spreads by skin-to-skin contact.

DIFFERENTIAL DIAGNOSIS

MC can be mimicked in immunocompromised patients by skin lesions of disseminated cryptococcosis, histoplasmosis, and other deep mycoses.

Figure 44–1 Molluscum contagiosum. A giant molluscum in a patient with acquired immunodeficiency syndrome (AIDS). Note the smaller, more typical lesion with central dell.

HOW TO MAKE THE DIAGNOSIS

The distinctive appearance of MC usually suffices. Direct examination of the whitish, curd-like content of the lesions mounted in 15% potassium hydroxide solution, or smeared on a slide and Giemsa-stained, shows the large intracytoplasmic inclusions characteristic of the disease ("molluscum bodies"). Atypical presentations in immunocompromised patients need punch or shave biopsy confirmation.

TREATMENT

Lesions that are few in number can be curetted easily. Anesthesia is seldom necessary. Cryotherapy with liquid nitrogen is effective. More aggressive treatment is indicated in immunocompromised patients. Laser ablation and electrodesiccation and curettage are the procedures of choice. Molluscum lesions have also been treated successfully by the application of the immune modifier imiquimod (5% cream) to the lesions each night for 4 weeks.

PROGNOSIS

For children, the prognosis is excellent. Resolution of MC even without treatment usually occurs in 3 to 9 months. For HIV-infected persons, the prognosis is guarded. Many cases are resistant even to aggressive treatment.

Chapter 45

CHERRY ANGIOMA
(ICD-9 228.01)

Lawrence Charles Parish

SYMPTOMS AND SIGNS

Cherry angiomas are asymptomatic lesions. Patients often become worried about the appearance of small (1 to 10 mm) red papules (Fig. 45–1). The lesions are benign and appear during early middle age, most commonly on the trunk.

A key clinical feature is the disappearance of the red color when direct pressure is applied, as viewed under a glass microscope slide, or when the surrounding skin is pulled taut.

DIFFERENTIAL DIAGNOSIS

Cherry angiomas are sometimes confused with insect bites or irritated seborrheic keratoses.

HOW TO MAKE THE DIAGNOSIS

The diagnosis of cherry angioma is clinical.

TREATMENT

The lesions are easily removed by snipping with an iris scissors followed by light electrodesiccation of the base or by cryosurgery.

Figure 45–1 Cherry angiomas. Small, red papules on the trunk that blanch with pressure.

PROGNOSIS

Cherry angiomas do not disappear on their own. Generally, a few form every year or so.

Chapter 46

GRANULOMA ANNULARE
(ICD-9 695.89)

Lawrence Charles Parish

SYMPTOMS AND SIGNS

Granuloma annulare (GA) is an asymptomatic condition. It begins as flat-topped to pinpoint firm red papules, 1 to 3 mm in diameter, which gradually enlarge to create a coin-like appearance (Fig. 46–1). The lesions are usually on the dorsal aspects of the hands and feet but may be found on the face, buttocks, ankles, wrists, and elbows. Sometimes, GA persists for several years and can involve most of the body—disseminated GA. Other forms of GA are rare: a plaque type that is flat and infiltrated, resembling necrobiosis lipoidica; an erythematous type that has red papules as the predominant morphology; a subcutaneous type that presents as subcutaneous nodules; and the perforans type, which ulcerates.

DIFFERENTIAL DIAGNOSIS

Annular GA may be confused with the annular form of sarcoidosis in which the lesions are predominantly facial, especially the nose. Tinea infections are scaling. Nodular GA on the elbows may be confused with rheumatoid nodules. Plaque GA resembles necrobiosis lipoidica.

Figure 46–1 Granuloma annulare. Red papules that gradually enlarge to coin-like lesions with raised borders.

HOW TO MAKE THE DIAGNOSIS

The diagnosis of GA is made by its characteristic clinical appearance. Confirmation may be obtained by the histopathologic examination of a punch biopsy specimen. Biopsy is the only way to diagnose the subcutaneous variety.

TREATMENT

Most therapy is minimally effective. Super-potent topical corticosteroid ointments or creams can be used. Topical immunomodulators are sometimes helpful, as is pentoxifylline 400 mg, thrice daily. The old adage that a biopsy makes the lesion disappear is stretching the truth.

PROGNOSIS

GA usually disappears within a few years, but it can last several years. It should not leave any scars.

Chapter 47

FOLLICULITIS
(ICD-9 704.8)

Lawrence Charles Parish

SYMPTOMS AND SIGNS

Folliculitis is asymptomatic and causes mild itching or tenderness. Although the follicular red papules and pustules can be found wherever there are hair follicles, the lesions are most often seen under the beard or on the neck, chest, back, buttocks, and thighs (Fig. 47–1). Occasionally, the inflammation is severe enough to create crusting and pain. This condition is an infection of the hair follicles. *Staphylococcus aureus* is the most common culprit. *Pseudomonas aeruginosa* is responsible for hot tub dermatitis. In this condition, the follicular lesions are predominantly on the trunk and buttocks.

DIFFERENTIAL DIAGNOSIS

Pustules from *Candida albicans* are distinguished by fungal cultures. Viral exanthems are usually accompanied by fever and other systemic manifestations.

HOW TO MAKE THE DIAGNOSIS

Folliculitis is a clinical diagnosis. Sometimes, it can be confirmed by a bacteriologic culture, although the pathogen is frequently not recovered.

Figure 47–1 Folliculitis. Mildly pruritic, erythematous follicular pustule.

TREATMENT

Because the inflammatory process is often minimal and the infection is superficial, topical antimicrobials such as mupirocin ointment 2% may be applied twice daily. Extensive skin disease or involvement of noticeably hairy areas requires 1 week of oral antibiotic therapy such as dicloxacillin, 250 mg three to four times daily, or erythromycin, 250 mg three times daily. An alternative antimicrobial is ciprofloxacin, 500 mg twice daily. Occasionally, washing with an antibacterial solution such as chlorhexidine 4% or applying benzyl peroxide 5% gel twice daily will stop the process. Using a low-potent topical corticosteroid lotion twice daily is another helpful approach.

PROGNOSIS

Folliculitis can usually be prevented by washing with soap. Avoiding occlusive lotions and pomades is the key to preventing folliculitis.

Chapter 48

PYOGENIC GRANULOMA
(ICD-9 686.1)

Lawrence Charles Parish

SYMPTOMS AND SIGNS

Pyogenic granuloma (PG) ranges from being asymptomatic to tender and painful. It may also bleed. Common sites are fingers, toes, lips, buccal mucosa, anal mucosa, and the upper aspects of the trunk. PGs measure 5 to 10 mm in diameter, are red to black (depending on trauma) and are often pedunculated, irritated, and friable (Fig. 48–1). PGs develop within a few weeks of injury to the site; they may also be caused by pregnancy or systemic retinoids. Despite the name, they are neither bacterial infections nor granulomatous, but are simply benign vascular hyperplasias. PGs are more common in children and young adults. They almost never involute spontaneously.

DIFFERENTIAL DIAGNOSIS

The clinical picture of PG is characteristic; however, an irritated nevus or seborrheic keratosis might be confused with a PG. Malignant melanoma may have the same appearance if it is pedunculated. Occasionally, an embedded tick may look like a PG.

HOW TO MAKE THE DIAGNOSIS

The history of easy bleeding and the clinical appearance of PG are usually sufficient for the diagnosis.

Figure 48–1 Pyogenic granuloma. A red, friable, pedunculated papule, which developed during pregnancy.

TREATMENT

A PG is easily removed by shaving the lesions and lightly electrodesiccating the base.

PROGNOSIS

Once a PG is removed, there should be no recurrence. The lesion itself does not cause scarring.

Chapter 49

MILIUM
(ICD-9 706.2)

John T. Crissey

SYMPTOMS AND SIGNS

Milium is a tiny asymptomatic keratinous cyst, the cause of which is unknown. Its clinical appearance is a round or oval, white or yellowish body directly beneath the surface of the skin. Milia are common. They occur singly or in groups and measure only 1 to 2 mm in diameter (Fig. 49–1). The cheeks, eyelids, forehead, temples, penis, scrotum, and the internal aspect of the labia minora are the favored sites. All age-groups are affected. Facial milia can be found in 50% of newborn infants; these lesions disappear spontaneously in a few weeks. Similar lesions in older children and adults sometimes disappear without treatment but usually persist indefinitely.

Milia may appear *de novo* or in association with the healing process of the lesions of other cutaneous problems, particularly vesiculobullous disorders—pemphigus vulgaris, epidermolysis bullosa, second-degree burns, porphyria cutanea tarda, bullous pemphigoid, and bullous lichen planus. Milia may also follow abrasions, radiation therapy, and dermabrasion.

DIFFERENTIAL DIAGNOSIS

The closed comedones of acne vulgaris sometimes resemble milia.

HOW TO MAKE THE DIAGNOSIS

The clinical appearance of milia is distinctive. Expression of the contents, a small whitish semisoft ball of keratinous debris, confirms the diagnosis.

Figure 49–1 Milium. Tiny, thin-walled papule filled with yellow keratin.

TREATMENT

The contents of milia are easily removed by opening the lesions with a cutting edge needle or a pointed scalpel blade and expressing the contents with a comedo extractor or by squeezing gently with the thumb and forefinger.

PROGNOSIS

Once removed, milia usually do not recur.

Chapter 50

SYRINGOMA
(ICD-9 M8407/0)

David H. Frankel

SYMPTOMS AND SIGNS

Syringomas are asymptomatic. Patients are often concerned about the cosmetic effect. Syringomas occur predominantly in women and begin during puberty. Most of them appear on the lower eyelids as 1 to 3 mm (in diameter), soft, white to yellowish translucent papules (Fig. 50–1). They usually occur in crops and may also appear on the cheeks and trunk.

DIFFERENTIAL DIAGNOSIS

Papules of acne vulgaris are erythematous and not usually limited to the lower eyelid. Dermatosis papulosa nigra (DPN) is a variant of the seborrheic keratosis that is most commonly found in darker-skinned patients. DPN may be quite numerous and extend from under the eyelids to the cheeks. Milia are pinpoint, thin-walled, white papules that appear and disappear spontaneously and are often seen on the upper eyelids.

HOW TO MAKE THE DIAGNOSIS

The diagnosis of syringoma is made by examination.

TREATMENT

Treatment is only for cosmetic purposes. Various destructive methods such as light electrodesiccation and laser ablation may be effective.

PROGNOSIS

Lesions will persist unless treated.

Figure 50–1 Syringoma. Tiny, translucent, white to yellow papules on the lower eyelids with crops of lesions under the left eye.

Chapter 51

FURUNCLE AND CARBUNCLE
(ICD-9 680.7) and (ICD-9 680.9)

John T. Crissey

SYMPTOMS AND SIGNS

Furuncles are painful and exquisitely tender. The cliché, "sore as a boil," is accurate. The furuncle is a *Staphylococcus aureus* infection seated deeply in a pilosebaceous unit. When two or more adjacent units are involved, the lesion is called a **carbuncle**. A firm erythematous nodule approximately 1 cm in diameter enlarges for several days, becomes fluctuant, points, and ruptures to drain a mixture of necrotic tissue and creamy pus streaked with blood (Fig. 51–1). Healing usually takes place in 1 or 2 weeks. A depressed saucer-like scar may result. Any area of the skin bearing hair follicles may be attacked, but the favored sites are areas subject to friction and sweating—buttocks, axillae, groin, face, and neck. In the carbuncle, initial redness and nodularity is more extensive. The lesion is larger, 6 to 8 cm in diameter. Pointing and drainage occur at several sites simultaneously. The carbuncle has a special predilection for the nape of the neck. Carbuncles heal much more slowly than furuncles.

DIFFERENTIAL DIAGNOSIS

Inflamed and ruptured epidermoid and pilar cysts sometimes resemble furuncles. The history of a preexisting nodule and the characteristic pasty,

Figure 51–1 Furuncle. Exquisitely tender, fluctuant, erythematous nodule in infected hair follicle.

rancid-smelling contents of these lesions serve to differentiate them from the furuncle or carbuncle. Early lesions of hidradenitis suppurativa may resemble furuncles.

HOW TO MAKE THE DIAGNOSIS

The clinical picture of a furuncle and a carbuncle is distinctive. Identification of the *Staphylococcus* in gram-stained smears or cultures of the pus establishes the diagnosis in atypical presentations.

TREATMENT

Incision and drainage of individual furuncles may suffice. Systemic antibiotics shorten the course and are mandatory in immunocompromised patients and in all patients with carbunculosis. Dicloxacillin and cephalexin are the medications of choice. A suitable dicloxacillin dosage schedule is 250 to 500 mg four times daily by mouth for 10 to 14 days. Cephalexin can be given in doses of 250 to 500 mg four times daily by mouth for 14 days. Recurrences in nasopharyngeal carriers can be minimized by the twice-daily intranasal application of mupirocin or bacitracin ointments. Failure to respond to the above schedules may indicate that the infection is caused by methicillin-resistant *S. aureus* (MRSA). Infections of this type have become increasingly common. They sometimes respond to oral clindamycin, but patients often require hospitalization and treatment with IV vancomycin. Resistant and recurrent cases may also merit a search for immune dysfunction.

PROGNOSIS

The prognosis is excellent in the absence of immunologic compromise.

Chapter 52

ERYTHEMA NODOSUM
(ICD-9 695.2)

John T. Crissey

SYMPTOMS AND SIGNS

Erythema nodosum (EN) is usually painful and tender. It is a reactive, inflammatory panniculitis that appears as indurated, erythematous nodules that can be single or multiple. The lesions are 1 to 20 cm in diameter and are hot to the touch. Older lesions often have a bluish, brownish, yellow–green, or purplish tinge and resemble contusions (Fig. 52–1). Borders are not sharply demarcated. Extensor surfaces of the lower leg, thigh, and ankle are the favored sites, although arms and other areas are occasionally affected. When multiple, EN nodules are usually bilateral, but not necessarily symmetric. Fever, arthralgia, and malaise may accompany or precede the eruption. The disease is much more common in women than men.

Most cases of EN occur in association with streptococcal infections or sarcoidosis. Behçet's syndrome, coccidioidomycosis, Crohn's disease, histoplasmosis, leprosy, lymphogranuloma venereum, lymphomata, psittacosis, pulmonary tuberculosis, and ulcerative colitis are also known causes, as well as medications, especially sulfonamides, iodides, and oral contraceptives. In many cases, the cause remains obscure.

The course of EN is variable. Lesions usually involute in a few weeks, but EN associated with chronic disease may persist or recur for many months.

Figure 52–1 Erythema nodosum. Painful nodules on the shins resemble contusions.

DIFFERENTIAL DIAGNOSIS

Cellulitis is usually not nodular, although pain and warmth are common. Insect bites, urticaria, lupus panniculitis, and erythema multiforme may be nodular and easily confused with EN.

HOW TO MAKE THE DIAGNOSIS

The clinical picture of EN is distinctive. Punch biopsy, deep enough to include subcutaneous fat, is indicated in atypical cases.

TREATMENT

Treatment should be directed against the cause, which must be searched for assiduously in every case. Bed rest, elastic bandages, and aspirin or nonsteroidal anti-inflammatory agents to tolerance are helpful. Injection of 0.1 to 0.5 mL of triamcinolone acetonide suspension, 5 mg/mL, directly into the nodules is a practical and effective approach when lesions are few in number. EN usually responds rapidly to systemic corticosteroids, but these agents are often contraindicated in the diseases that cause the eruption. Saturated solution of potassium iodide by mouth, five to six drops three times daily for 2 to 3 weeks, is sometimes remarkably effective.

PROGNOSIS

Prognosis is good when the underlying disease can be controlled. Recurrences are common in idiopathic EN.

Chapter 53

HIDRADENITIS SUPPURATIVA
(ICD-9 705.83)

John T. Crissey

SYMPTOMS AND SIGNS

In hidradenitis suppurativa (HS), painful, tender, erythematous, nodular lesions appear in the axillary, genital, and perianal areas (Fig. 53–1). Open comedones and patulous follicular orifices in and about the inflammatory areas are hallmarks of the disease. HS usually begins at a single site, but eventually appears in other apocrine gland-bearing areas as well. In severe cases, the buttocks, thighs, periumbilical areas, nipples, and scalp may be involved. Nodules suppurate, point, rupture, and drain pus, blood, and serous exudates. Sinus tracts form. Scarring is prominent. The disease progresses in fits and starts. HS is due to recurrent bacterial infection of apocrine glands (apocrine acne) and is primarily a disease of young adults. HS is sometimes associated with cystic acne vulgaris, occasionally with pilonidal sinuses or with Crohn's disease.

Figure 53–1 Hidradenitis suppurativa. Painful, tender nodules in apocrine areas such as the axilla.

131

DIFFERENTIAL DIAGNOSIS

Initial acutely inflamed lesions of HS are indistinguishable from furunculosis. The short course and complete resolution of the latter serve to differentiate the two conditions. The deep mycoses, scrofuloderma, lymphogranuloma venereum, and granuloma inguinale (donavanosis) may all mimic HS.

HOW TO MAKE THE DIAGNOSIS

The diagnosis of HS is made clinically. The long history of recurrences and the presence of scarring is especially helpful.

TREATMENT

The choice of systemic antibiotics for treating HS is guided by results of culture and sensitivity. *Staphylococcus aureus* is the organism primarily responsible for HS. However, multiple antibiotics may be necessary when *S. aureus*, streptococci, *Escherichia coli, Proteus*, or *Pseudomonas* strains are also isolated. Isotretinoin in the doses employed in the treatment of cystic acne vulgaris, has also been used with some success in the treatment of hidradenitis in its early stages. Intralesional injections with triamcinolone acetonide are definitely helpful. A dose of 0.1 to 0.3 mL of a 5 to 10 mg/mL suspension can be injected into nonfluctuant sites every 2 or 3 weeks for several months. Incision and drainage of fluctuant nodules are indicated. Excision of fibrotic nodules and sinus tracts is often successful. Intractable disease involving large areas may require complete excision and skin grafting.

PROGNOSIS

Prognosis is good for control, but less promising for cure. HS tends to diminish and may even involute completely as the patient approaches middle age.

Chapter 54

CHONDRODERMATITIS NODULARIS CHRONICA HELICIS
(ICD-9 380.0)

John T. Crissey

SIGNS AND SYMPTOMS

Tenderness is the hallmark of chondrodermatitis nodularis chronica helicis (CNCH). Patients pull away when the lesion is touched, and they are often awakened at night when they roll over and the pillow comes into contact with the area. Some lesions are subject to sudden episodes of intense pain not associated with contact of any kind. CNCH is a chronic disease of the skin of the ear, which presents as one or several small, dome-shaped, skin-colored, or erythematous papular excrescences, usually at the apex of the helix or anthelix (Fig. 54–1). An adherent scale overlying a central horny plug is evident in the typical lesion. The right ear is more often involved than the left. CNCH is largely a disease of the middle-aged and elderly. Men are more commonly affected than women. The cause is thought to be localized trauma from excessive telephone use, earphones, head bands, and the like, although clear-cut evidence for such is seldom present.

DIFFERENTIAL DIAGNOSIS

Molluscum contagiosum lesions, verruca vulgaris, actinic keratoses, and the tophi of gout may resemble CNCH. None of these approach CNCH in lesional tenderness.

HOW TO MAKE THE DIAGNOSIS

The history, location, appearance, and tenderness of the lesions combine to render this an easy diagnosis. Histopathology is characteristic. When doubt exists, a punch or shave biopsy can be diagnostic.

TREATMENT

Removal of sources of trauma is indicated when they are known. Excision, desiccation and curettage, and ablation with carbon dioxide and argon lasers, have all been used with success. Intralesional injections with an insoluble corticosteroid such as triamcinolone acetonide are sometimes effective; 0.1 to 0.3 mL of a 5 to 10 mg/mL suspension can be injected into the base of the lesion once a month for 2 or 3 months.

PROGNOSIS

The prognosis is good, but recurrences are common after all forms of treatment.

Figure 54–1 Chondrodermatitis nodularis chronica helicis. Painful papule on the helix of the ear.

Chapter 55

KELOID AND HYPERTROPHIC SCAR
(ICD-9 701.4) and (ICD-9 701.4)

John T. Crissey

SYMPTOMS AND SIGNS

Both hypertrophic scars and keloids have a tendency to itch; keloids are sometimes tender and painful. They are overgrowths of fibrous tissue at the sites of trauma or inflammatory disease processes. Keloids and hypertrophic scars present as firm papular or nodular lesions. The shoulders, upper trunk, ear lobes, chin, neck, and the lower part of the legs are the favored sites.

Keloids begin in a site of trauma, but continue to grow for prolonged periods of time, often extending many centimeters beyond the initial site to form large elevated mesa-like plaques (Fig. 55–1). Keloids may also appear as knobby individual lesions, dome-shaped nodules that resemble cobblestones, or irregular shiny plaques from which ridge-like bands and cords extend like pseudopods. The surface may be reddish or purplish at first and later hyper or hypopigmented. Lesions located over joints can seriously interfere with

Figure 55–1   Keloid extending far beyond point of ear piercing.

135

function. Keloid susceptibility is sometimes familial; the condition is more common in dark-skinned individuals.

Hypertrophic scars tend to follow the shape of original trauma, such as linear incisions, suture tracks, and circumscribed burn areas. They usually reach a certain size and stop growing.

DIFFERENTIAL DIAGNOSIS

Fibromata, pigmented basal cell carcinomata, and the skin lesions of sarcoidosis sometimes resemble keloids.

HOW TO MAKE THE DIAGNOSIS

Location and morphology point to the proper diagnosis. A punch biopsy confirms the clinical diagnosis if doubt exists. In many instances, differentiation between keloid and hypertrophic scars can only be made after extended observation.

TREATMENT

No completely satisfactory treatment is available. Intralesional injections with an insoluble corticosteroid, such as triamcinolone acetonide suspension, are helpful in softening lesions and relieving pain and tenderness. A dose of 0.1 to 0.3 mL of a 20-mg/mL suspension can be injected into several lesional sites once a month for 3 or 4 months. Cryotherapy with liquid nitrogen is useful for smaller lesions. Results with laser ablation are encouraging. Surgical excision of ear lobe keloids is often successful, but the excision of lesions in other areas is usually followed by prompt recurrence unless combined with adjuvant treatments such as radiation, compression, or intralesional corticosteroids. The application of imiquimod (5% cream) to the surgical site daily for several weeks after the excision of keloids may discourage recurrences. Similarly, application to surgical wound sites in keloid-prone patients may be helpful in keloid prevention. The prolonged application of silicone sheets postoperatively to surgical wounds in patients with a tendency to develop keloids or hypertrophic scars has also been helpful.

PROGNOSIS

Prognosis is good for improvement with treatment, but poor for a totally satisfactory result. Some keloids and hypertrophic scars diminish in size with the person's age. Patients should be aware that unnecessary procedures, whether medical or otherwise, may result in avoidable lesions.

Chapter 56

LIPOMA
(ICD-9 214.9)

John T. Crissey

SYMPTOMS AND SIGNS

Lipomas are asymptomatic in most cases, although larger lesions that impinge on nerves are sometimes painful. A lipoma presents as a palpable, ill-defined, sometimes lobulated, soft or doughy mass, a "miniature pillow beneath the skin" (Fig. 56–1). Lipomas are mobile and not fixed to the overlying skin. They are common and usually make their initial appearance in early middle age. The size varies. Most are small, 2 or 3 cm in diameter, although lesions of long duration can be many centimeters in diameter.

Growth is slow. The neck, shoulders, and back are the most common sites involved, but no area is exempt. The skin overlying the lesion is normal in appearance, and occasionally slightly pigmented. Lipomas are usually solitary or few in number, although they occur in large numbers in familial multiple lipomatosis, an autosomal dominant condition. This condition usually begins in early adulthood.

DIFFERENTIAL DIAGNOSIS

Deep-seated epidermal inclusion cysts sometimes mimic lipomas.

Figure 56–1 Lipoma. Soft, doughy mass under the skin.

HOW TO MAKE THE DIAGNOSIS

Location, mobility, and consistency point to the proper diagnosis. Needle aspiration biopsy confirms the diagnosis in doubtful cases.

TREATMENT

Total excision is curative, although not necessary for these benign lesions. Large lipomas associated with deeper anatomic structures may be difficult to excise. Liposuction has been successful in the eradication of smaller lesions.

PROGNOSIS

Lipomas are benign and remain so. Most stabilize at some point and stop enlarging.

Chapter 57

XANTHELASMA
(ICD-9 272.2)

John T. Crissey

SYMPTOMS AND SIGNS

Asymptomatic flat or slightly raised, yellow to yellow–orange plaques appear on the eyelids, particularly on the nasal side (Fig. 57–1). Small at first, the lesions slowly enlarge, and in some cases progress to involve virtually the entire lid. Most patients with xanthelasma are middle-aged or older. Xanthelasma in patients younger than 30 years is usually a sign of significant disturbances in lipoprotein metabolism. In approximately 60% of patients, xanthelasma is a normolipoproteinemic xanthoma with no demonstrable systemic cause. Nevertheless, these lesions may be associated with hyperlipoproteinemias that can result in atherosclerotic cardiovascular disease.

DIFFERENTIAL DIAGNOSIS

Eyelid milia of unusual size can resemble the lesions of xanthelasma.

HOW TO MAKE THE DIAGNOSIS

The location and distinctive color combine to confirm the diagnosis of xanthelasma. All patients with xanthelasma should be checked for hyper-lipoproteinemia.

TREATMENT

The lesions can be treated successfully with electrodesiccation, excision, carbon dioxide laser ablation, or careful application of 35% trichloroacetic acid solution.

Figure 57–1 Xanthelasma. Yellow plaques on lower eyelids.

PROGNOSIS

The prognosis is excellent in normolipoproteinemic cases, guarded when associated with hyperlipoproteinemia.

Chapter 58

XANTHOMA
(ICD-9 272.2)

John T. Crissey

SYMPTOMS AND SIGNS

Xanthomata are asymptomatic lesions. The most important of these lesions commonly encountered in practice are those associated with genetically-based disturbances in lipoprotein metabolism, namely, the familial forms of hypercholesterolemia, dyslipoproteinemia, combined hyperlipoproteinemia, and hypertriglyceridemia. Xanthelasma (see Chapter 57) and arcus senilis, a gray ring at the periphery of the cornea, are sometimes seen in these disorders. Palpable and visible lesions appear in several distinctive forms.

Eruptive xanthomata appear suddenly as crops of small, asymptomatic, discrete, dome-shaped papules on the buttocks and thighs. The arms, elbows, knees, and palms may also be involved. Reddish at first, the lesions soon take on a yellowish or yellowish–brown color (Fig. 58–1). Some are surrounded by a reddish halo. The papules may run together to form plaques. **Eruptive xanthomata** may occur in hyperlipoproteinemias secondary to other metabolic diseases, especially poorly controlled diabetes mellitus.

Xanthoma tendinosum presents as firm, nontender, subcutaneous nodules associated with tendons. The Achilles and patellar tendons, and extensor tendons of the hands are the favored sites. Overlying skin is usually normal in appearance, occasionally yellowish.

Figure 58–1 Eruptive xanthoma appear as red papules that become yellow or yellow–brown with time.

Xanthoma tuberosum presents as smooth, nontender, yellowish papules and nodules on the elbows and knees.

Xanthoma striatum palmare lesions are yellow to yellow–orange infiltrations along the palmar and digital flexural creases, often accompanied by papular xanthomata on the palms.

DIFFERENTIAL DIAGNOSIS

Keloids resemble old, tuberous lesions in darker-skinned patients but are preceded by trauma. Cutaneous sarcoid is usually more waxy in appearance, but may be indistinguishable.

HOW TO MAKE THE DIAGNOSIS

The yellow color and characteristic morphology usually permit the diagnosis of xanthoma to be made at sight. Punch biopsy findings are distinctive and confirm the clinical diagnosis when doubt exists.

TREATMENT

Management depends on the exact nature of the causative metabolic disturbance. A complete lipid workup is essential. Therapy includes dietary restrictions, weight control, and pharmacologic measures to control lipid levels.

PROGNOSIS

Xanthomata usually respond satisfactorily to treatment. Early recognition and control of the underlying metabolic disturbances can also significantly reduce the incidence and severity of cardiovascular problems with which the genetic lipoprotein disturbances are closely linked.

Chapter 59

WARTS
(ICD-9 078.1)

John T. Crissey

SYMPTOMS AND SIGNS

Warts are generally asymptomatic. They are caused by human papilloma virus (HPV) infections of the skin and mucocutaneous surfaces. All lesions are potential sources of infection. They appear in several different forms.

Verruca Vulgaris

Verruca vulgaris is the common wart that usually occurs on the hands, fingers, wrists, and forearms of children and young adults. Nail folds are often involved. No area is immune to infection. The lesions are asymptomatic, flat or dome-shaped papules, 2 to 10 mm in diameter (Fig. 59–1). They may run together to form still larger lesions. Early verrucae are usually smooth. Mature lesions are rough; the surface becomes covered with tiny keratotic projections. Warts may be skin-colored, yellowish, brown, or dark gray. They sometimes occur in linear configurations, the virus having been inoculated in a scratch "like planting a row of potatoes" (Koebner's phenomenon).

Verruca Plantaris (Plantar Warts)

Unlike other verrucae, plantar lesions are often tender and sometimes painful. They usually appear at the pressure points on the sole, where callus formation often obscures the true nature of the lesion. Trimming the callus reveals a whitish sodden circle studded with dark red or black dots (thrombotic capillaries), a sign that is virtually diagnostic. Larger lesions may also show evidence of pressure-induced intralesional hemorrhage. Multiple plantar verrucae may run together to produce mosaic-like patterns, sometimes involving almost the entire sole.

Figure 59–1 Verruca vulgaris on the finger.

Figure 59–2   Verruca plana. Smooth, brown, flattened papules are often on the face.

Verruca Plana (Flat Warts)

Verruca plana are usually seen on the face or dorsum of the hands in young people. They are skin-colored, pinkish or brownish, sharply marginated, flat papules, 1 to 3 mm in diameter (Fig. 59–2). The surface of the papules is relatively smooth. The lesions are discrete, scattered irregularly or distributed in groups. Linear configurations (Koebner's phenomenon) are common.

Verruca Filiformis

Filiform verrucae are single or multiple, small, slender, thread-like projections with a frayed keratotic tip. They usually occur on the eyelids, nares, and other parts of the face, occasionally on the neck.

Condyloma Acuminatum

Condylomata acuminata present as exuberant, pink to red, moist, papular warts on mucocutaneous surfaces, particularly the genitalia, perianal area, and crural folds (Fig. 59–3). They bleed easily and are often foul-smelling. Lesions on adjacent skin surfaces may assume the clinical form of verruca vulgaris. Condylomata are usually contracted through sexual contact. They spread rapidly in pregnancy. Several of the strains of the HPV that cause condylomata predispose patients to cervical dysplasia, cervical, vulvar, anal, or penile squamous cell carcinoma. In children, condylomata are sometimes a sign of sexual abuse.

DIFFERENTIAL DIAGNOSIS

Skin tags can mimic verruca filiformis. Large callouses can be mistaken for verruca plantaris. Condyloma latum lesions of secondary syphilis sometimes resemble condyloma acuminatum.

HOW TO MAKE THE DIAGNOSIS

Most forms of verrucae are diagnosable at sight from the morphology alone. Trim the callus over plantar lesions and look for the characteristic black

Figure 59-3   Condyloma acuminata on the penis.

dots. Histopathology is distinctive; punch or excision biopsy can confirm the clinical diagnosis in atypical presentations.

TREATMENT

No true antiviral therapy is available. All active treatment is an assault designed to ablate the virus and its captive host tissue completely or stimulate a favorable immune response. Assault techniques commonly used include liquid nitrogen cryotherapy, light electrodesiccation, curettage, laser ablation, and application of salicylic acid plasters.

    When few in number, condylomata acuminata are best treated with electrodesiccation. For more extensive cases, topical applications of podophyllin, podofilox, or imiquimod are useful. A 15% to 25% solution of podophyllin in compound tincture of benzoin is applied to the condylomata and washed off in 2 hours. To avoid excessive reaction, treatment should be confined to a 5 to 6 cm^2 area at each sitting. Applications can be repeated at weekly intervals. Podofilox gel 5%, a podophyllin relative marketed in kits, can be applied at home by the patient. Podofilox is applied with a cotton-tipped swab every 12 hours for 3 consecutive days and then withheld for 4 days. These cycles can be repeated four times. Podofilox is contraindicated in pregnancy. Imiquimod, marketed as a 5% cream, is applied sparingly to the condylomata by the patient three times per week at bedtime and washed off with soap and water 6 to 10 hours later. It is continued until a satisfactory result is obtained, but for no more than 16 weeks.

    Imiquimod (5% cream) has now been approved for the treatment of condylomata acuminata. The cream should be applied three times per week to the cleaned wart area at bedtime, and should remain on the skin for 6 to 10 hours. Treatment should continue until there is clearance of visible genital or perianal warts, or for a maximum of 16 weeks. Uncircumcised men treating warts under the foreskin should retract the foreskin and wash the area daily. Similarly, the treatment of verruca vulgaris and verruca plana has also been successful, although not in all cases.

Prompt gynecologic consultation is indicated when condylomata appear on the genitalia during pregnancy. Infants delivered vaginally in this situation can develop recurrent respiratory papillomatosis in later life.

PROGNOSIS

Most verrucae eventually disappear whether treated or not. Condylomata acuminata are less likely to do so.

Section V

Spots

Chapter 60

KAPOSI'S SARCOMA
(ICD-9 176.0)

Jeffrey P. Callen

SYMPTOMS AND SIGNS

No specific symptoms are associated with Kaposi's sarcoma (KS). KS occurs in two forms—one related to aging (classic form) and another due to immune suppression (acquired or iatrogenic). The classic form most often occurs on the legs and consists of violaceous patches, papules, or plaques (Fig. 60–1). This form is more prevalent in persons of Mediterranean and/or Jewish ancestry. KS associated with immunosuppression occurs in any site and is often mistaken for a simple ecchymosis. KS is a vascular neoplasm associated with human herpesvirus-8 infection.

Figure 60–1 Classic Kaposi's sarcoma presenting as nonblanching violaceous patches and papules on the lower extremities.

DIFFERENTIAL DIAGNOSIS

Ecchymoses are not papular or indurated. Neither are telangiectasias. Bacillary angiomatosis must be considered in differential diagnosis, particularly in the human immunodeficiency virus (HIV)-infected individual.

HOW TO MAKE THE DIAGNOSIS

Punch biopsy confirms the diagnosis. Systemic KS should be excluded by a chest roentgenogram and computed tomography of the abdomen.

TREATMENT

In the elderly patient with classic KS, therapy with local irradiation or destruction with liquid nitrogen is often effective. Vinblastine or other antineoplastic agents are used for systemic disease. For immunosuppressed patients, therapy should aim to improve immune function. Patients with HIV-associated KS often respond to combinations of newer antiretroviral therapies. For organ transplantation patients, the condition often remits as immunosuppressive therapy is eased; however this can result in the loss of the transplanted organ. A recent study detailed the disappearance of KS in organ transplant patients without a loss of organ function when cyclosporin and/or mycophenolate were replaced by sirolimus.

PROGNOSIS

Patients with classic KS and localized disease have an excellent prognosis. In immunosuppressed patients or patients with disseminated disease, death due to this neoplasm is possible from bleeding, infection, or dysfunction of vital organs.

Chapter 61

ECCHYMOSIS/ACTINIC PURPURA
(ICD-9 459.89)/(ICD-9 287.2)

Jeffrey P. Callen

SYMPTOMS AND SIGNS

Ecchymoses are asymptomatic or tender nonpalpable hemorrhages, usually 1 cm or more in diameter. They usually follow trauma, even mild trauma. The lesions are often linear or angulated and tend to occur on the dorsal hands, extensor forearms, pretibial area, and anterolateral thighs. The most common form of ecchymotic hemorrhage, actinic purpura, occurs on the sun-damaged skin of the elderly (Fig. 61–1).

DIFFERENTIAL DIAGNOSIS

Considerations for differential diagnosis include deficiencies of vitamin C or vitamin K, disseminated intravascular coagulopathy, leukemia, immune thrombocytopenic purpura, hemophilia, Kaposi's sarcoma, Ehlers–Danlos

Figure 61–1   Actinic purpura on the sun-damaged skin of the forearm.

syndrome, von Willebrand's disease, and anticoagulant, corticosteroid (systemic or topical), and aspirin therapy. Domestic violence must also be considered.

HOW TO MAKE THE DIAGNOSIS

Clinical examination is usually sufficient for the diagnosis of ecchymosis/actinic purpura. Biopsy is rarely necessary. The history should assess the use of drugs and dietary habits. Laboratory testing, if necessary, should include platelet count, prothrombin time, partial thromboplastin time, and bleeding time.

THERAPY

No treatment is needed for actinic purpura. Vitamin K–containing creams are of unproven benefit. Prevention of trauma may help prevent further lesions. Treatment of any underlying conditions may reverse the process.

PROGNOSIS

Ecchymoses are benign and usually resolve within weeks.

Chapter 62

CUTANEOUS VASCULITIS
(ICD-9 446.20)

Jeffrey P. Callen

SYMPTOMS AND SIGNS

Patients with vasculitis may complain of burning or pain in the affected areas. The condition is often accompanied by systemic involvement, manifested as arthralgias, myalgias, fever, abdominal pain, or hematochezia. Palpable purpura is the most common cutaneous sign (Fig. 62–1). However, urticarial lesions, ulcerations, nodules, or livedo reticularis (a bluish discoloration in a net pattern) can also occur. Palpable purpura or urticarial lesions are more common in small blood vessel disease, whereas medium-sized vessel involvement manifests as livedo reticularis, nodules, or ulcers. Vasculitis may be a sign of many underlying conditions, including infections (e.g., bacterial endocarditis, acute respiratory infections, or hepatitis B or C), drug reactions (from aspirin, penicillin, sulfonamides, or others), cryoglobulinemia, collagen vascular disorders (e.g., systemic lupus erythematosus, rheumatoid arthritis, or Sjögren's syndrome), lymphoproliferative disorders, and Henoch–Schönlein purpura.

DIFFERENTIAL DIAGNOSIS

Patients with purpuric lesions from cholesterol emboli often have a history of recent angiography. Capillaritis or thrombocytopenia causes purpura that is nonpalpable. Urticarial vasculitis is an unusual condition that should be suspected when individual lesions persist beyond 24 hours. Insect bite reactions and physical urticarias must also be considered.

Figure 62–1 Cutaneous vasculitis with palpable purpura due to ampicillin.

HOW TO MAKE THE DIAGNOSIS

The diagnosis of cutaneous vasculitis is confirmed by punch biopsy. The best site for biopsy is a fresh lesion, preferably less than 24 hours old. When assessing the possibility of medium-sized vessel involvement, a deeper and larger biopsy is often required. In patients with an obvious cause, testing is directed toward determining systemic involvement: renal function tests, urinalysis, and chest x-ray. In patients without an identifiable cause, the laboratory assessment should include blood cultures (in patients with fever), paraproteins, cryoproteins, hepatitis C virus antibody, antinuclear antibody, antineutrophil cytoplasmic antibody (ANCA), rheumatoid factor, and serologies for lupus erythematosus and Sjögren's syndrome.

TREATMENT

Therapy for cutaneous vasculitis ranges from observation with symptomatic therapy to aggressive immunosuppressive agents. Drug-associated vasculitis usually resolves when the offending agent is withdrawn. Patients with chronic cutaneous vasculitis may respond to oral colchicine, 0.6 mg twice daily; dapsone, 100 to 200 mg daily; low-dose methotrexate, 10 to 25 mg weekly; or azathioprine, 1 to 2 mg/kg daily. Systemic corticosteroids may be useful, but steroid-related toxicity is common, and whenever possible these agents should be avoided. Patients with hepatitis C–associated vasculitis may be treated effectively with antiviral regimens including interferon-α-2a, 3 million units subcutaneously three times per week, and ribavirin, 1,000 to 1,200 mg per day orally for 24 to 48 months. Henoch–Schönlein purpura is treated symptomatically. Rituximab has been demonstrated to be useful in ANCA-associated vasculitis.

PROGNOSIS

The prognosis of cutaneous vasculitis is dependent on the degree of systemic involvement and the severity of the underlying diseases.

Chapter 63

POSTINFLAMMATORY HYPOPIGMENTATION
(ICD-9 709.00)

Jeffrey P. Callen

SYMPTOMS AND SIGNS

Generally, postinflammatory hypopigmentation is asymptomatic unless there is still an existing inflammatory disorder elsewhere. Patients with darker skin are more prone to develop this condition. The inflammatory reaction that precedes this may be intense and obvious, or it may be subtle and even barely noticed by the patient. The problem is a common sequela of eczema (Fig. 63–1). Mild atopic dermatitis can result in pityriasis alba, hypopigmented patches on the face most commonly seen in African-American children. Hypopigmentation frequently follows cutaneous lupus erythematosus, both in chronic and subacute forms, and lichen planus.

DIFFERENTIAL DIAGNOSIS

Vitiligo is due to total loss, not simply a decrease, in pigmentation. Under the Wood's lamp, its border is sharply defined, and there is no pigmentation. Postinflammatory hypopigmentation is ill defined, and there is evidence of incomplete pigment loss.

Figure 63–1 Postinflammatory hypopigmentation due to eczema.

HOW TO MAKE THE DIAGNOSIS

Postinflammatory hypopigmentation can usually be diagnosed on clinical examination. Punch biopsy is helpful at times in determining the cause of the hypopigmentation.

TREATMENT

Therapy for the causative condition of postinflammatory hypopigmentation aids in the prevention of additional lesions. In many cases, the pigmentation returns. But generally, darker patients take longer to repigment. Because pityriasis alba causes subtle continued inflammation, a low- to medium-potent topical corticosteroid may be helpful.

PROGNOSIS

Postinflammatory hypopigmentation has, by itself, no implied prognosis. The prognosis is directly linked to the disease that caused it.

Chapter 64

LICHEN SCLEROSUS ET ATROPHICUS
(ICD-9 701.0)

Jeffrey P. Callen

SYMPTOMS AND SIGNS

Patients with lichen sclerosus et atrophicus (LS&A) complain of rough or dry patches of skin that are sometimes pruritic (Fig. 64–1). Genital lesions cause sexual dysfunction and dyspareunia. LS&A presents commonly as kraurosis vulvae, a keyhole or "figure 8" configuration of well-demarcated, hypopigmented, slightly atrophic patches around the vulva and perineum (Fig. 64–2). Skin atrophy is common; the surface is shiny and wrinkles like cigarette paper. Lesions on the penis are called **balanitis xerotica obliterans**.

DIFFERENTIAL DIAGNOSIS

At times, LS&A overlaps with morphea (localized scleroderma) in the same patient. Genital lesions of lichen planus are often violaceous and erosive and are accompanied by lesions on the skin or mucous membranes or both. The possibility of sexual abuse is considered when hemorrhage occurs in genital lesions.

HOW TO MAKE THE DIAGNOSIS

Clinical suspicion of LS&A is confirmed by punch biopsy.

Figure 64–1 Generalized lichen sclerosus in an elderly woman.

Figure 64–2 Lichen sclerosus et atrophicus. Kraurosis vulvae with "keyhole" configuration around the vulva and perineum.

TREATMENT

Despite the fact that LS&A appears to be an atrophic process, super-potent topical corticosteroid ointments are highly effective. When topical steroids are used on the genitalia, topical anticandidal therapy may also be needed to prevent secondary yeast infection. Topical testosterone has been used in the past, but this therapy is ineffective and often associated with androgenic toxic effects. Therefore, it should be discarded as a potential therapy. Topical calcineurin inhibitors such as pimecrolimus or tacrolimus might be useful but should probably be avoided on genital lesions.

PROGNOSIS

Some patients have spontaneous resolution of LS&A, particularly children. It appears that genital lesions may be associated with subsequent development of squamous cell carcinoma, and this is the reason that I avoid calcineurin inhibitors on this area.

Chapter 65

VITILIGO
(ICD-9 709.1)

Jeffrey P. Callen

SYMPTOMS AND SIGNS

Vitiligo is usually asymptomatic, but because the depigmented skin is very sensitive to sunlight, patients may complain of sunburn (Fig. 65–1). Periorificial depigmentation is observed early in the course (Fig. 65–2). Acral areas are commonly affected. Depigmented areas are sharply demarcated from adjacent, normally pigmented skin. Vitiligo can occur at any age, but most commonly during adolescence or young adulthood. The disease is believed to be the result of an autoimmune disorder that targets the melanocyte, and it is not uncommon for patients to have associated autoimmune disorders, such as thyroiditis, pernicious anemia, and alopecia areata.

DIFFERENTIAL DIAGNOSIS

In postinflammatory hypopigmentation, there is usually a history of a preexisting inflammatory skin disorder such as eczema or lichen planus. Wood's light examination demonstrates only partial loss of pigment. Piebaldism is congenital, localized, and nonprogressive, and there are multiple color variations. Hydroquinone-containing products and some other chemicals can cause pigment loss.

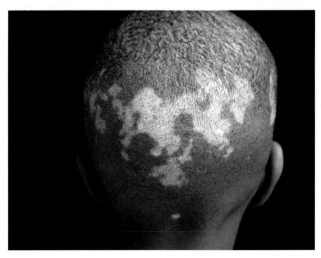

Figure 65–1 Vitiligo. Depigmentation on the scalp.

Figure 65–2   Periorificial vitiligo showing sharp demarcations between normally pigmented and depigmented skin.

HOW TO MAKE THE DIAGNOSIS

The diagnosis of vitiligo is clinical. Punch biopsy is rarely needed. After the diagnosis is established, patients should be assessed for associated conditions through thyroid function tests and a complete blood count.

TREATMENT

Medium- or high-potent topical corticosteroid ointments or creams may be effective. Although vitiliginous skin seems less prone to atrophy from topical steroids, reevaluation should be done every 4 to 6 weeks and include a Wood's light examination. Therapeutic response is usually noted within 2 to 3 months and often begins in a perifollicular pattern. Topical tacrolimus or pimecrolimus have been demonstrated to be effective. PUVA therapy, ultraviolet A (UVA) light combined with oral or topical psoralen—a photosensitizing agent—is another approach. This therapy is administered two to three times weekly in a controlled setting under the direction of a physician. Narrowband ultraviolet B (UVB) phototherapy might also be effective in many patients, and localized treatment with this type of light delivered by a laser is also potentially useful for patients with localized disease. It often takes 6 to 8 weeks for phototherapy-based treatments to begin to take effect. Sending patients to tanning facilities is not advisable.

PROGNOSIS

Vitiligo is difficult to treat. Because the skin lacks pigments, it is more prone to sunburn. Therefore, sun protection methods and sun blocks should be used. Patients should be assessed for skin cancer regularly.

Chapter 66

MORPHEA (LOCALIZED SCLERODERMA)
(ICD-9 701.0)

Jeffrey P. Callen

SYMPTOMS AND SIGNS

Morphea (localized scleroderma) is an asymptomatic condition limited to the skin. Some patients complain of a tight feeling of their skin, or pruritus or burning. Morphea is a localized hardening of the skin. The condition occurs in three forms—plaques, linear, and generalized. Plaques of morphea are indurated and red to violaceous at the borders (Fig. 66–1). Linear scleroderma has a similar appearance. It occurs on the face, where it is known as "*en coup de sabre*," or on the extremities. Facial linear scleroderma may rarely affect underlying tissues including the bones and the brain and is known as **Parry–Romberg syndrome**. In generalized morphea, the plaques are large and widespread.

DIFFERENTIAL DIAGNOSIS

Localized scars usually have a history of trauma. Systemic scleroderma (progressive systemic sclerosis) is characterized by sclerodactyly, Raynaud's phenomenon, and systemic involvement, which is manifested as dysphagia, arthritis, and dyspnea.

Figure 66–1   Morphea. Extensive hyperpigmented and violaceous plaques.

HOW TO MAKE THE DIAGNOSIS

The diagnosis of morphea is clinical, but it is useful to perform a punch biopsy for confirmation. Laboratory abnormalities are relatively uncommon in localized scleroderma, with the exception of a positive antinuclear antibody test (40% to 50%) and, frequently, the presence of antihistone antibodies (25% to 50%).

TREATMENT

There is no uniformly accepted therapy for morphea. In fact, it is not clear whether any of the proposed therapies work. Patients with overlapping features of lichen sclerosus et atrophicus may respond to super-potent topical corticosteroid ointments or creams. Topical calcipotriene cream or ointment 0.005% once or twice daily applied under occlusion has been reported to be effective. Topical tacrolimus or pimecrolimus might also be effective. Several studies have demonstrated methotrexate with or without systemic corticosteroids to be effective. Physical therapy helps patients with joint deformities.

PROGNOSIS

Over a period of months to years, most patients have spontaneous softening of affected areas. Those with facial hemiatrophy may be left with permanent disfigurement, and those with lesions occurring over joints may have contractures.

Chapter 67

SCLERODERMA (PROGRESSIVE SYSTEMIC SCLEROSIS)
(ICD-9 710.1)

Jeffrey P. Callen

SYMPTOMS AND SIGNS

The onset of scleroderma [progressive systemic sclerosis (PSS)] is insidious. Patients often complain first of Raynaud's phenomenon. In this condition the skin is taut and bound down and is shiny and may become dyspigmented. The disease may be limited or diffuse. The limited form of PSS is more common and is characterized by a slowly progressive hardening of the acral skin, a condition known as **sclerodactyly** (Fig. 67–1). In diffuse PSS, sclerodactyly is accompanied by widespread involvement of both the skin and the internal organs. The systemic symptoms include fatigue, dysphagia, dyspnea, abnormal bowel function, arthralgias, and myalgias. Hypertension may be caused by PSS involving the kidneys. A variant, known as the **CREST syndrome**, is characterized by *c*alcinosis, *R*aynaud's phenomenon, *e*sophageal dysmotility, *s*clerodactyly, and *t*elangiectasia.

Figure 67–1   Scleroderma. Sclerodactyly; taut, bound-down skin on hands.

DIFFERENTIAL DIAGNOSIS

Morphea (localized scleroderma) is a distinct and separate disease causing localized areas of induration. Eosinophilic fasciitis (EF), which is rare, causes a rapid onset of proximal sclerosis without associated Raynaud's phenomenon. Patients with EF have eosinophilia and hyperglobulinemia. The clinical manifestations characteristically begin after an episode of excessive exertion. Eosinophilia–myalgia syndrome has features similar to those of EF but is triggered by contaminated L-tryptophan.

HOW TO MAKE THE DIAGNOSIS

Scleroderma is diagnosed by a constellation of findings after the exclusion of other diseases. Once diagnosed, the patient should be assessed for the severity of the disease. Laboratory evaluation includes serologic tests for antinuclear antibodies, anticentromere antibody (ACA), and antitopoisomerase I (Scl-70) antibody. The ACA is common in patients with the CREST variant (80% to 90%). Scl-70 indicates diffuse and often rapidly progressive PSS. Patients also should undergo esophageal motility studies if they complain of dysphagia and, if they have other gastrointestinal symptoms, upper gastrointestinal x-rays with bowel follow-through. Chest x-ray and pulmonary function tests should be performed in all patients because of the high rate of asymptomatic pulmonary dysfunction.

TREATMENT

There is no cure for PSS. It is not clear whether the process can be arrested or reversed. The use of D-penicillamine and extracorporeal photopheresis is controversial. Nonspecific therapy is directed at the symptoms and signs, for example, calcium channel blockers (e.g., nifedipine 30 to 60 mg daily by mouth) or topical nitroglycerin for Raynaud's phenomenon, nonsteroidal anti-inflammatory drugs for arthralgias and myalgias, and elevation of the head during sleep to prevent aspiration in patients with esophageal dysmotility.

PROGNOSIS

The prognosis for patients with PSS is dependent on the presence of systemic disease. Although patients with renal involvement represent less than 5%, approximately 30% to 50% of them have rapidly progressive and life-threatening disease. In the absence of renal disease, scleroderma is slowly progressive, and the presence and severity of cardiopulmonary involvement determines the outcome. Survival of patients with the CREST variant can be 10 to 20 years in the absence of progressive pulmonary dysfunction.

Chapter 68

LENTIGO
(ICD-9 709.0)

Charles A. Gropper

SYMPTOMS AND SIGNS

Lentigines are asymptomatic small, brown macules. There are three major types: lentigo simplex, solar lentigo, and lentigo maligna.

Lentigo simplex may occur anywhere on the skin or mucous membranes. It is a small macule, approximately 1 to 8 mm in diameter, tan to dark brown or black in color, and uniformly pigmented. Lentigo simplex is not related to sun exposure. In Peutz–Jeghers syndrome, simple lentigines are associated with polyps of the gastrointestinal tract and increased risk of gastrointestinal or genitourinary carcinoma (Fig. 68–1).

Solar lentigo, known by the lay term "liver spot," has a similar appearance to that of lentigo simplex, but is induced by sunlight. It develops on the sun-exposed areas, usually in older people, and can be larger than lentigo simplex, up to 2 cm in diameter.

Lentigo maligna is a large brown patch with irregular pigmentation and shape on the sun-damaged skin (Fig. 68–2). It is most common in patients older than 60 years. Approximately 5% of lentigo malignas progress to lentigo maligna melanomas; they are therefore sometimes referred to as "malignant melanoma *in situ.*"

DIFFERENTIAL DIAGNOSIS

Unlike freckles, lentigines do not darken with sunlight and can occur anywhere on the body, including the mucous membranes. Junctional nevi can appear identical to lentigines on examination and sometimes can only be differentiated on biopsy. Nevi and flat seborrheic keratoses frequently have a bumpy surface. Pigmented actinic keratoses occur on the sun-damaged skin and are red and scaling. Lentigo maligna must be distinguished from

Figure 68–1 Simple lentigo on the lips of a patient with Peutz–Jeghers syndrome.

Figure 68-2 Lentigo maligna with irregular borders and variable pigmentation on the sun-exposed skin (one lesion).

lentigo maligna melanoma by punch or excisional biopsy. Lentigo maligna appears on the sun-damaged skin and has markedly irregular pigmentation and irregular borders. Lentigo maligna melanoma has similar findings, but variability of color and border irregularity are more pronounced.

HOW TO MAKE THE DIAGNOSIS

The diagnosis of lentigines is often clinical, but excisional biopsy must be done if malignant melanoma is suspected.

TREATMENT

Lentigo simplex and solar lentigines are treated mainly for cosmetic reasons. Lentigines that are very dark in color should be biopsied to rule out melanocytic atypia. Lentigo simplex and solar lentigo can be treated with cryotherapy, tretinoin cream 0.025% daily, or surgical excision. The use of sunscreens and sun avoidance can be helpful for solar lentigines.

Surgical excision is the most effective treatment for lentigo maligna, but more conservative treatments such as cryotherapy or electrodesiccation and curettage may be sufficient. Several types of newly developed lasers have been used in the treatment of lentigos. The Q5 Nd!YAG laser and the ruby laser are effective in the treatment of solar lentigo and lentigo simplex. The ruby laser also has been reported to be effective in the treatment of lentigo maligna; however, surgical removal remains the most definitive treatment.

PROGNOSIS

Lentigo simplex and solar lentigines are benign lesions. They usually persist throughout life, although a small number will fade or disappear. In contrast, lentigo maligna is a lesion with known premalignant potential. Malignant degeneration of lentigo maligna usually occurs in lesions that have been present for more than 10 years. Because approximately 5% of lentigo maligna lesions will progress to lentigo maligna melanomas, they must be followed closely with a bias toward early biopsy and treatment.

Chapter 69

POSTINFLAMMATORY HYPERPIGMENTATION
(ICD-9 709.00)

Charles A. Gropper

SYMPTOMS AND SIGNS

Patients with postinflammatory hyperpigmentation often complain of an asymptomatic dark spot or patch on the skin that seemed to appear "out of nowhere." The spot may have blurred borders and may be irregularly shaped (Fig. 69–1; Fig. 2–2). Because any inflammatory dermatosis can heal with hyperpigmentation, the diagnosis of this condition is suggested by the history of a preceding rash that has evolved into a darker hue in the same distribution. Patients are often concerned that the darkening of color indicates a worsening of their condition; they need reassurance that the color change is actually a part of the healing process.

HOW TO MAKE THE DIAGNOSIS

The diagnosis of postinflammatory hyperpigmentation is established by the history of prior inflammatory dermatosis and clinical appearance.

DIFFERENTIAL DIAGNOSIS

Melasma appears in a symmetric distribution on the cheeks and is frequently associated with pregnancy. In acanthosis nigricans, the skin surface is usually bumpy and scaly, and the condition is limited to the axillae, posterior neck, and groin. Patients who have used bleaching creams with hydroquinones can develop exogenous ochronosis characterized by intensely dark patches on the

Figure 69–1 Postinflammatory hyperpigmentation due to eczema.

affected areas. Tinea versicolor is a common yeast infection of the skin that presents with slightly hyperpigmented scaly plaques on the chest and back; this condition often heals with hypopigmentation. Erythema dyschromicum perstans, also known as ashy dermatosis, is a rare condition characterized by round, hyperpigmented, slightly scaly plaques occuring most often on the trunk.

TREATMENT

Identification and treatment of the inflammatory dermatosis that caused the hyperpigmentation is an important first step. Treatment is difficult; it is hard to predict which patients will respond and how well they will respond. There are several treatment options, all of which are most helpful if applied within the first 2 months of the development of hyperpigmentation.

Bleaching creams containing 4% hydroquinone may be effective if the pigmentation is very superficial and confined to the epidermis. Alternatives include high-potent topical corticosteroid ointments or creams applied daily or tretinoin cream 0.05% applied each night. Patients should be encouraged to use sun block with sun protection factor (SPF) of at least 15 to decrease the chances of further hyperpigmentation due to sunlight.

PROGNOSIS

Postinflammatory hyperpigmentation may take months or years to disappear.

Leg Ulcers

Chapter 70

LEG ULCERS
(ICD-9 707.1)

John T. Crissey

SYMPTOMS AND SIGNS
Venous Ulcers (Stasis Ulcers)

Venous ulcers are more common in women; patients are usually middle-aged or older, often with a history of thrombophlebitis. Although pain and tenderness associated with venous ulcers may be pronounced, symptoms are usually less prominent than one might expect from the clinical appearance. Venous ulcers often follow a minor injury. They are usually unilateral, involving the lower third of the leg and ankle, especially the malleoli. The borders are sharp and often irregular. The surrounding skin may be markedly thickened, hyperpigmented, and pebbly. Chronic lymphedema is also often present. The base of the ulcer, which bleeds easily when disturbed, is made up of granulation tissue and necrotic slough in varying proportions (Fig. 70–1).

Signs of chronic venous insufficiency in the areas surrounding the ulcers provide clues to the diagnosis: red–brown speckles of hemosiderosis against the more uniformly brownish background of hyperpigmentation, along with scattered purpuric macules. Eczematous changes—patchy areas of brighter erythema, moist papules, scaling, serous crusting, and excoriations—may also be present.

Arterial Ulcers (Ischemic Ulcers)

Atherosclerosis is the usual cause of arterial ulcer (AU) in the elderly. Men are more susceptible than women. AUs are uncommon before middle life. Pain is the outstanding feature, and intermittent claudication is often prominent. Arterial ulcers are usually sharply defined and round, as if punched out (Fig. 70–2). They tend to be smaller than venous ulcers and may be deep enough to expose muscle and tendons. The base is commonly covered with a necrotic slough. Pretibial areas, toes, and dorsa of the feet are the favored sites.

Changes in the skin of the legs, ankles, and feet provide clues to the diagnosis of AU. There is pallor and often cyanosis, sometimes accompanied by the mottled violaceous erythema known as livedo reticularis. The pallor is especially evident when the leg is elevated. Changes are usually bilateral. The legs and feet have a cold, clammy feel. Thickening and distortion of the toenails (onychogryphosis) and the absence of arterial pulses are common signs as well.

Figure 70–1 Venous stasis ulcer on lower leg with bleeding, granulation tissue with surrounding venous stasis changes.

Figure 70–2 Arterial ulcer with sharp borders in a patient with poor circulation due to diabetes.

DIFFERENTIAL DIAGNOSIS

When leg ulcers occur in the absence of either venous or arterial insufficiency, the cause is usually a bacterial infection preceded by a traumatic episode. Ulcers belonging to this group can be located anywhere on the leg and are seldom more than 3 or 4 cm in diameter. They are usually tender and are often surrounded by a prominent zone of erythema. Bacterial and fungal cultures are indicated when vascular problems are absent. Punch biopsy of the border of the lesion is helpful in these cases. Special stains can be used to identify fungi and other microorganisms or to identify neoplastic disease, which is also an occasional cause. Streptococci, staphylococci (especially enterococci), mycobacteria, *Treponema pallidum,* and *Leishmani donovani* are all capable of producing ulcers on the legs. The punched-out ulcers about the ankles characteristic of sickle cell disease usually occur in younger patients, who show no signs of venous or arterial insufficiency.

HOW TO MAKE THE DIAGNOSIS

Note the history and morphology, check for circulatory problems, and culture and biopsy the ulcer border if circulation appears normal. Biopsy material should be stained for bacteria and fungi.

TREATMENT

Treatments of venous ulcers are largely strategies for improving venous return: leg elevation, elastic stockings and roll bandages, and surgical intervention (ligation and stripping procedures). Grafting is sometimes feasible. Eczematous eruptions (stasis dermatitis) usually improve with medium, high or super-potent topical corticosteroid ointments or creams.

For arterial ulcers, the long-range goal is to eliminate or control as many of the major risk factors associated with peripheral vascular disease as possible, namely smoking, hypertension, hyperlipoproteinemia, obesity, and diabetes mellitus. Foot care is of great importance. Corns, callosities, and nail dystrophies merit professional attention. Pharmacologic treatment, although often disappointing, is worth trying. Pentoxifylline has produced beneficial results in some cases at a dosage of 400 mg three times daily by mouth (with meals). Surgical consultation is indicated in every case. Distal arterial bypass grafting or lumbar sympathectomy may offer the best or only chance to preserve a severely compromised extremity.

The treatment of leg ulcers that are not circulatory in origin must be tailored to the cause.

PROGNOSIS

Venous ulcers tend to be chronic. Compliance with therapy and preventive measures can significantly improve prognosis. Prognosis in arterial ulcers is guarded. Surgical intervention offers the best hope for a successful outcome.

Section VII

Nails and Nail Folds

Chapter 71

ONYCHOMYCOSIS
(ICD-9 110.9)

Charles A. Gropper

SYMPTOMS AND SIGNS

Onychomycosis is usually asymptomatic. Sometimes, however, it is painful, especially when there is a secondary bacterial infection or when the dystrophic growth pattern causes an ingrown toenail. In a small number of extremely severe cases, there can be difficulty in ambulation. Affected nails become yellow, thickened, and onycholytic, meaning that the nail plate partially separates from the nail bed (Fig. 71–1). Toenails are more often affected than fingernails; one common pattern is the infection of both feet, but only one hand. It is common for only some nails on a foot or hand to be involved, whereas neighboring nails are spared.

Onychomycosis is extremely common. Total prevalence in the United States is in the range of 5% to 10%, and up to 20% of individuals over the age of 40 will have this problem at some point in their lives. The most common agent is *Trichophyton rubrum.*

DIFFERENTIAL DIAGNOSIS

Psoriatic nails can appear identical with nails with onychomycosis, with yellowing, hyperkeratosis, and onychocholysis. Psoriatic nails may have additional clinical features such as pitting and "oil spots," which are yellow–brown spots

Figure 71–1 Yellow, thickened, and onycholytic toenails due to *Trichophyton rubrum.*

under the nail plate. The presence of typical psoriatic plaques on other parts of the body suggests the diagnosis of psoriasis.

HOW TO MAKE THE DIAGNOSIS

The clinical diagnosis of onychomycosis can be confirmed by identifying fungal elements in a 10% potassium hydroxide preparation of nail plate scales. Alternatively, nail clippings may be sent to the laboratory for fungal culture, but results take weeks to arrive. A nail clipping can also be sent to the dermatopathology lab for periodic acid-Schiff (PAS) stain for fungal organisms. None of these tests is positive in 100% of the cases, so a clinical impression must be the final arbiter of diagnosis.

TREATMENT

Until recently, the mainstay of treatment for onychomycosis was at least 1 year of therapy with griseofulvin. Even then, the success rate was only approximately 30%, and the relapse rate was over 50%. The availability of the two new oral agents, terbinafine and itraconazole, has greatly improved treatment options. Terbinafine, 250 mg daily, is given for 6 weeks for fingernails and 12 weeks for toenails. Itraconazole can be given as a "pulse dose," in which the patient takes 200 mg twice daily for 1 week of each month. This regimen is followed for 2 months for fingernails and 3 months for toenails. Liver function tests should be checked before either treatment and rechecked 1 month after treatment begins.

Topical antifungal preparations are much less effective than systemic treatment for onychomycosis because much less medication successfully penetrates the nail plate. However, for patients who are unable or unwilling to take systemic medications, there is a U.S. Food and Drug Administration (FDA)-approved (ciclopirox 8% topical solution) topical lacquer for nail fungus. It is applied each night to the toenails. Clinical studies with this medication showed 12% of patients with a complete cure and 36% with significant improvement.

PROGNOSIS

With terbinafine and itraconazole, onychomycosis is cured in approximately 80% of patients. Patients must be reminded that nail growth is slow. The full effect of treatment is not seen until 6 to 8 months in fingernails and 9 to 12 months for toenails. The relapse rate is approximately 15% within 18 months of treatment.

Chapter 72

PSEUDOMONAS NAILS
(ICD-9 041.7)

Charles A. Gropper

SYMPTOMS AND SIGNS

Patients with *Pseudomonas aeruginosa* infection of the nail plate complain of blue–green changes or of a sickly sweet, "fruity" smell similar to that of rotting grapes (Fig. 72–1). The blue–green pattern may occur in sequential transverse bands reflecting intermittent intensity of infection. Sometimes, the paronychial areas swell. In general, this is an indolent condition. This problem occurs in individuals whose hands are frequently wet.

DIFFERENTIAL DIAGNOSIS

Dermatophyte infections turn nails yellow.

HOW TO MAKE THE DIAGNOSIS

The diagnosis of *Pseudomonas* nails is made on the basis of the characteristic appearance and odor. The culture of involved nail plates sometimes confirms the diagnosis. The submission of a nail specimen for pathologic examination is less helpful because *Pseudomonas*, unlike fungus or yeast, is difficult to identify in the nail plate during pathologic examination.

Figure 72–1 Green nails due to *Pseudomonas aeruginosa* infection.

TREATMENT

Nails usually respond rapidly to topical or systemic antibiotics that offer good gram-negative coverage. A good choice is ciprofloxacin, 750 mg twice daily by mouth for 10 days.

PROGNOSIS

Fingernails will appear normal for 3 to 6 months after the active infection has been eradicated. For toenails, the wait may be twice as long.

Chapter 73

ACUTE AND CHRONIC PARONYCHIA
(ICD-9 112.3) and (ICD-9 681.02)

Charles A. Gropper

SYMPTOMS AND SIGNS

Acute paronychia is a very painful and tender infection of the proximal and lateral nail folds. It is usually caused by *Staphylococcus aureus*; occasionally, group A streptococci, and gram-negative bacteria are responsible. The nail folds become red and swollen, and there may be frank drainage of pus (Fig. 73–1). After several months, the nail may break (onycholysis) or become ridged. Acute paronychia frequently occurs in diabetics and in patients who are immunocompromised.

Chronic paronychia has a less dramatic presentation and is often due to *Candida albicans*. Contact dermatitis, fixed drug eruptions, psoriasis, and dyshidrotic eczema also cause chronic paronychia. Repeated hand trauma or washing leads to a loss of the seal between the nail plate and nail folds, and infectious or irritative agents can gain entry. Dentists, bakers, and construction workers are often affected.

DIFFERENTIAL DIAGNOSIS

Nail-folds welling and erythema of herpetic whitlow often extends to the finger, and Tzanck smear or viral culture confirms the diagnosis. Neoplasms of the nail matrix are usually painless. Careful examination shows a narrow band of alteration of the nail plate, reflecting the focal location of the lesion within the nail matrix. A history of psoriasis or eczema, along with characteristic lesions on other parts of the body suggests these diagnoses.

Figure 73–1 Acute paronychia with tender, red, swollen proximal and lateral nail folds.

HOW TO MAKE THE DIAGNOSIS

The significant pain and the clinical appearance of paronychia make the diagnosis. Culture may demonstrate responsible organisms.

TREATMENT

Severe, painful, acute paronychia may require lancing with a No. 11 blade to release the purulent fluid accumulating under the nail fold. Patients who require lancing should always be treated with antistaphylococcal antibiotics for at least 7 days. In chronic paronychia due to *Candida*, lancing is not indicated. Topical therapy, such as imidazole cream (see Chapter 23) or 2% to 4% thymol in chloroform (or absolute alcohol) two to three times daily may suffice. In severe cases, an oral agent such as itraconazole, 200 mg daily for 7 days, may be necessary. Because chronic paronychia is often superinfected with bacteria, a course of antistaphylococcal antibiotics may also be necessary.

PROGNOSIS

The infection tends to be recurrent, especially in patients who are unable to avoid frequent hand washing. Patients can be advised to wear light cotton gloves under their work gloves. They should also avoid direct contact with irritants, where possible. Resolution of nail changes may take up to 6 months after an infection is resolved.

ALOPECIA AREATA
(ICD-9 704.01)

Charles A. Gropper

SYMPTOMS AND SIGNS

In alopecia areata (AA), round patches of hair loss develop rapidly and asymptomatically. The patches are well-circumscribed, round, and without inflammation or scarring (Fig. 74–1). Hair loss occurs most commonly on the scalp, but other areas such as the eyebrows and beard are often involved. AA is a chronic, recurrent condition that often begins in childhood or in young

Figure 74–1 Alopecia areata. Patches of alopecia are well-circumscribed, round, and without inflammation.

adults. The term **alopecia totalis** is used if all scalp hair is lost, and **alopecia universalis** is the term for complete loss of all body hair. As much as 1% of the population may have at least one spot of AA by age 50. There is a positive family history of AA in 10% to 20% of patients.

One pathognomonic sign of AA is the "exclamation point" hair, which is wide distally and narrow at the base and occurs at the periphery of a patch of hair loss (Fig. 74–2). Hairs that regrow in a patch of AA are often white. Pitting of the nails accompanies hair loss in approximately 40% of patients. Most patients are in good health, and no additional medical workup is required. In a small number of cases, however, there is an association with other autoimmune conditions such as Hashimoto's thyroiditis, connective tissue disease, myasthenia gravis, cataracts, and vitiligo.

DIFFERENTIAL DIAGNOSIS

In tinea capitis, there is scaling and erythema. Trichotillomania appears in an irregular-shaped patch of hair loss, not well circumscribed as in AA, with some of the hairs having broken ends. The patient may also have a history of hair trauma and petechiae on the scalp around follicles. Androgenetic alopecia involves most of the scalp rather than small round patches and occurs in characteristic male or female patterns.

Figure 74–2 Alopecia areata. Exclamation point hairs are wide distally and narrow at the base.

HOW TO MAKE THE DIAGNOSIS

The presence of well-demarcated, round patches of nonscarring alopecia is characteristic. Exclamation point hairs and nail pitting, when present, are helpful in confirming the diagnosis of AA (Fig. 74–2). Punch biopsy is usually not needed to rule out other causes.

TREATMENT

AA has a variable course, and new lesions may develop even as old ones are resolving. This makes the evaluation of treatments difficult, and no treatment has been extremely effective. The main treatment option in AA is intralesional injection of dilute glucocorticosteroids such as triamcinolone acetonide suspension in a concentration of 2.5 to 5 mg/mL. The injections are given every 3 to 4 weeks. The total dose per treatment session should not exceed 20 mg. Topical corticosteroid ointments or creams may be used as an additional treatment, but efficacy is marginal. It is best to use high-potent topical corticosteroids, although the results are marginal. These steroids can be used for weeks to months, but skin atrophy is a concern with prolonged use. Topical anthralin, which elicits a mild contact immune response, has been used with modest success. The cream is applied nightly, in a concentration starting at 0.1% and increasing to 1% as tolerated. Minoxidil solution 2% or 5% is of mild benefit in some patients.

PROGNOSIS

Approximately 33% of patients with AA have complete hair regrowth within 1 year. Eighty percent of patients who first develop this condition after puberty eventually have complete regrowth. Complete regrowth is even more assured in children. Poor prognostic signs include the involvement of the occipital region, repeated attacks, nail changes, and total alopecia before puberty.

Chapter 75

ANDROGENETIC ALOPECIA
(ICD-9 704.00)

Charles A. Gropper

SYMPTOMS AND SIGNS

Androgenetic alopecia is asymptomatic but often causes great psychological distress. Hair loss is gradual, and there are no surface changes on the scalp. The hairs become shorter and narrower and eventually fall out. In men, the frontotemporal scalp and vertex are most commonly involved, and progression to complete hair loss may occur. In general, hair density decline approximately 15% before it is noticed.

Women also experience androgenetic alopecia. Unlike in men, however, the pattern is more diffuse, although hair loss on the crown is common (Fig. 75–1). The pattern of hair loss in androgenetic alopecia in women has been described as resembling a christmas tree in which the top of the tree points toward the back of the scalp, and the region of hair loss widens toward the front of the scalp; the edges of the area of hair loss are uneven and wavy, much like the branches of a tree. Women only rarely develop male-pattern frontotemporal alopecia, and complete hair loss is rare.

DIFFERENTIAL DIAGNOSIS

It is helpful in any case of hair loss to distinguish between scarring and nonscarring diseases. Examine the follicles carefully. Scarring alopecia is characterized by disruption of follicles, in some cases with crust, erosion, or

Figure 75–1 Diffuse hair loss in a woman with androgenetic alopecia.

thickening of the scalp. The presence of scarring alopecia suggests diagnoses such as lupus erythematosus or dissecting cellulitis. Nonscarring alopecia points toward medical causes of hair loss, such as androgenetic alopecia, telogen effluvium, alopecia areata, and thyroid dysfunction. Medications causing alopecia include oral contraceptives, coumarin, heparin, propranolol, and vitamin A.

Telogen effluvium tends to involve the entire scalp uniformly and follows a period of stress by 3 to 6 months. Alopecia areata presents with well-circumscribed, round patches of hair loss. Secondary syphilis appears as a patchy, "moth-eaten" alopecia and should be associated with other findings, such as scaly rash, mucous patches, and condyloma latum.

HOW TO MAKE THE DIAGNOSIS

The diagnosis of androgenetic alopecia is made by the history of gradual, progressive loss of hair in the characteristic distribution. Punch biopsy is usually not necessary to confirm the diagnosis.

TREATMENT

For men, two treatments are now available, which have limited benefit. Minoxidil solution, 2% or 5% applied twice daily, results in decrease of hair shedding in approximately 80% of patients. Up to 60% of patients experience at least minimal regrowth of hair within 12 months of commencing treatment. With finasteride, 1 mg daily by mouth, 80% of men will have the same or a greater amount of hair after 2 years of therapy, and 65% will have at least some visible regrowth. The drug may cause decreased libido, erectile dysfunction, and ejaculation disorders in approximately 2% of patients.

For women, minoxidil solution 2% applied twice daily brings results similar to those seen in men. Finasteride is contraindicated in women; it is dangerous for pregnant women to touch the pills because of a risk of genital malformations in the fetus.

PROGNOSIS

Progression of androgenetic alopecia is unpredictable.

Chapter 76

TELOGEN EFFLUVIUM
(ICD-9 704.02)

Charles A. Gropper

SYMPTOMS AND SIGNS

Telogen effluvium is asymptomatic. Hair loss in telogen effluvium is evenly distributed throughout the scalp. Approximately 30% to 50% of the scalp hair is involved, so patients do retain a fairly full head of hair even during the worst of the shedding process (Fig. 76–1). There is no scarring. Sometimes referred to as telogen defluvium, the condition is a sudden diffuse loss of scalp hair occurring 3 to 6 months after a stressful event, such as systemic illness or pregnancy. The hair loss is caused by the simultaneous cycling of an unusually high percentage of scalp hairs into the resting, or telogen, phase. Normally, approximately 5% to 10% of hairs are in the telogen phase; during telogen effluvium, this number increases to approximately 30%. Normally, resting hairs are retained in the scalp for approximately 80 to 100 days until they are shed. This explains the 3- to 6-month delay in the development of clinically apparent hair loss after the stressful event. Additional causes of telogen effluvium include neoplasms, infections, and crash diets. Some medications have also been implicated, including heparin, coumarin, propanolol, haloperidol, and lithium.

Chronic telogen effluvium is a recently described variant in which patients, typically women aged 30 to 60 years, develop the sudden onset of diffuse hair shedding on the scalp without an obvious precipitating event. Unlike classic telogen effluvium which usually resolves within a few months,

Figure 76–1 Telogen effluvium after pregnancy.

chronic telogen effluvium may persist for many years. In this condition, patients continue to shed hairs but do not become bald, because they continue to produce new hairs.

DIFFERENTIAL DIAGNOSIS

In androgenetic alopecia or alopecia areata, the areas of hair are well circumscribed and not diffuse in contrast to telogen effluvium.

HOW TO MAKE THE DIAGNOSIS

The diagnosis of telogen effluvium is suggested by the history of a recent stressful event. A hair pull test reveals greater than normal numbers of telogen hairs with clubbed ends. In patients with telogen effluvium, approximately 50% of hairs have the clubbed ends; in healthy patients, only 10% of hairs are clubbed.

TREATMENT

No treatment is needed for telogen effluvium apart from reassurance.

PROGNOSIS

In most cases, there is complete regrowth of hair within a few months.

Procedures and Supplies

Chapter 77

PUNCH BIOPSY

David J. Leffell

Equipment needed
- Antiseptic solution
- 1% lidocaine with/without 1:100,000 epinephrine solution
- 20% aluminum chloride hexahydrate solution
- Biopsy punch (1 to 10 mm diameter)
- Iris scissors
- Nonabsorbable suture
- Needle driver
- Syringe and needle
- Sterile bandage
- Antibiotic ointment
- Tissue pathology bottle with formalin

CONSIDERATIONS

Punch biopsy is most helpful in diagnosing skin conditions whose characteristic pathology lies in the dermis. It is the best biopsy technique for undiagnosed rashes and suspected neoplasms.

PROCEDURE

- Prepare the lesion and surrounding skin with antiseptic solution.
- Anesthetize the site with lidocaine 1% with or without epinephrine (1:100,000). Do not use epinephrine on the digits or on the tip of the penis. It is safe, however, on the nasal tip and ears. Epinephrine can reduce bleeding and make visualization of the lesion easier. The anesthetic effect may be almost immediate, but it is best to wait 3 to 5 minutes before proceeding with the biopsy. The full hemostatic effect takes somewhat longer to occur and helps to maintain hemostasis after the procedure.
- Select the proper punch size. The size depends on the size of the lesion, how much of the lesion (or dermatitis) must be removed to make the histologic diagnosis, its anatomic location, and the differential diagnosis. Punches of 3 and 4-mm diameter are used most often. Disposable punches are reliably sharper than reusable instruments.
- Gently pinch the skin around the lesion at various angles to determine the direction that the skin stretches and compresses most easily (Fig. 77-1A).
- Traction should be placed along the axis that was most easily pinched (i.e., perpendicular to the relaxed skin tension lines; Fig. 77-1B).
- Place the punch atop the lesion and perpendicular to the skin.

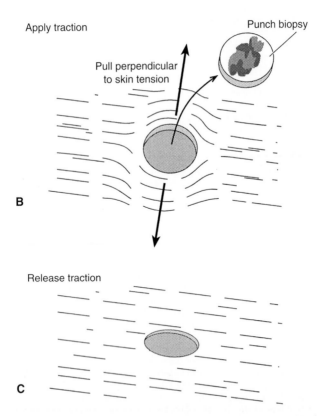

Figure 77–1 Punch technique, oval wound. **A:** Determine direction that the skin around the lesion stretches and compresses most easily. **B:** Apply tension in direction opposite skin tension lines (*arrows* in direction of tension). **C:** Punch biopsy defect becomes easily sutured oval shape after relaxation of tension.

- Advance the punch firmly with a gentle pushing and twisting motion that can be clockwise or counterclockwise. As the punch descends through the dermis and into the fat, a "give" is felt as tissue resistance decreases. It is very important to not remove the punch periodically to check the progress or depth. This traumatizes the tissue and may cause histologic artifact.
- Remove the punch only after it enters the fat. Release traction and observe how the circular defect becomes oval and more amenable to suturing (Fig. 77-1C).
- Lift the tissue sample using a single-prong skin hook or a needle (such as the one used for local anesthesia). The sample must not be crushed or artifact will result.
- Cut the base of the column of tissue with a pair of fine-curved iris scissors, and place the sample in formalin solution in the sample bottle for transport to the pathology laboratory. Be sure to give your dermatopathologist the patient's pertinent history, a description of the lesion, and the differential diagnosis.
- Apply pressure, hemostatic gauze, aluminum chloride solution (or place sutures) to control bleeding. Small defects can heal by second intention, but most wounds heal more rapidly and with a better cosmetic result if closed with simple interrupted or vertical mattress sutures.
- Close the wound. Typically two sutures close a 3- to 4-mm punch biopsy defect.
- Cover the wound with an antibiotic ointment such as polymyxin/bacitracin and a simple sterile dressing.
- Remove sutures on the face in 4 to 7 days. Remove sutures on the trunk in 5 to 7 days; sutures on the extremities should be removed in 7 days.

WOUND CARE INSTRUCTIONS TO PATIENTS

After 24 hours, patients should clean the wound gently with soap and tap water daily. Showering is fine as long as the wound is protected and kept dry.

Chapter 78

SHAVE BIOPSY AND SHAVE EXCISION

David J. Leffell

Equipment needed
- Antiseptic solution
- 1% lidocaine with/without epinephrine 1:100,000 solution
- 20% aluminum chloride hexahydrate solution
- Sterilized carbon steel razor blade (cut in half lengthwise)
- Cotton-tipped applicator
- Sterile bandage
- Bacitracin/polymyxin ointment

CONSIDERATIONS

Shave biopsy is most helpful in diagnosing diseases where the pathology is in or near the epidermis. Lumps and bumps, as opposed to rashes, are best biopsied with the shave technique. Such lesions appear pedunculated, papular, or exophytic. These include seborrheic keratoses, warts, intradermal nevi, pyogenic granulomas, actinic keratoses, basal cell carcinomas, and squamous cell carcinomas. Lesions suspected of being melanoma should not be biopsied in this manner.

PROCEDURE

- Prepare the lesion and surrounding skin with antiseptic solution.
- Mark the lesion with a sterile marking pen (anesthesia may blur the outlines).
- Anesthetize the site with lidocaine 1% with or without epinephrine (1:100,000). Do not use epinephrine on the digits or on the tip of the penis. It is safe, however, on the nasal tip and ears. Epinephrine can reduce bleeding and make visualization of the lesion easier. The anesthetic effect may be almost immediate but it is best to wait 3 to 5 minutes before proceeding. The full hemostatic effect takes somewhat longer to occur and helps maintain hemostasis after the procedure.
- Hold the flexible, half-razor blade between the thumb and middle or index finger, and remove the lesion with a gentle, forward sawing motion. The depth of excision is determined by the arc of the blade. Note that the blade arc is controlled by pressure placed on the ends of the blade (Fig. 78–1).
- Hold down the specimen with the wooden end of a cotton-tipped applicator. This prevents the incompletely removed lesion from flipping away from the blade.
- Place the specimen in formalin and send it to the laboratory. Be sure to give the dermatopathologist the patient's pertinent history, a description of the lesion, and a differential diagnosis.
- Remove any remnants of tissue at the margin of the biopsy by scraping it with a curette, with the belly of a No. 15 blade, or with the edge of the razor blade.

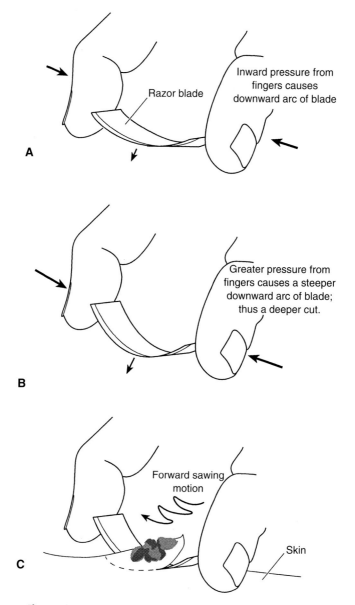

Figure 78–1   A–C: Depth of shave is adjusted by arc of half-razor blade.

- Apply pressure, or 20% aluminum chloride solution, or both. Avoid iron-containing styptics such as 20% ferric subsulfate (Monsel's solution) on the face. They can cause permanent tattoos.
- Apply antibiotic ointment, and dress the wound with a sterile bandage.

WOUND CARE INSTRUCTIONS TO PATIENTS

Patients should be advised to clean the wound with tap water and apply antibiotic ointment and a new bandage daily. Keeping wounds open to the air and allowing crust formation retards healing. A moist, occluded wound heals quicker and with less pain.

Chapter 79

CRYOSURGERY

David J. Leffell

Equipment needed
- Liquid nitrogen
- Liquid nitrogen reservoir (20- to 30-L flask)
- Paper or polystyrene cup
- Pressurized spray canister
- Spray tips and probes of various sizes for canister
- Cotton-tipped applicators, various sizes
- Otoscope speculums or neoprene cones

CONSIDERATIONS

Cryosurgery is the therapeutic application of cold, a "controlled frostbite." Many different cryogens have been used. Liquid nitrogen, at a temperature of $-195.8°C$ ($-320.4°F$), is the most common. Cryosurgery effectively treats many superficial lesions, such as actinic keratoses, lentigines, molluscum contagiosum, seborrheic keratoses, and warts. Deeper, malignant lesions such as basal cell carcinoma are also treated with cryotherapy, but this requires special equipment and expertise and is not as successful as other methods.

Cryosurgery causes intracellular and extracellular ice crystal formation, alterations in tissue, and vascular stasis. These changes lead to tissue anoxia and necrosis. Melanocytes are most easily destroyed by cryosurgery. This means that hypopigmentation can be a permanent complication of therapy, especially in dark-skinned patients. However, lentigines, for example, can be eliminated without harming the keratinocytes or dermis. Moreover, because fibroblasts are relatively insensitive to cold, scarring rarely follows the treatment of superficial lesions.

Cryosurgery can be performed by applying liquid nitrogen with cotton-tipped swabs or by spraying it with the use of a pressurized canister (Fig. 79–1). For either technique, a fast freeze and a slow thaw cause the greatest amount of tissue damage. The extent of tissue damage depends on the pressure, duration of application, and the number of freeze-thaw cycles.

PROCEDURE

Application Technique

- Tease and twist the end of a cotton-tipped swab so that it is no more than 1 to 2 mm larger than the lesion being treated.
- Dip the swab into the cup of liquid nitrogen, and then hold it firmly against the lesion.
- For thin lesions (such as actinic keratoses and lentigines), 5 to 10 seconds of firm contact should cause formation of an ice ball 1 to 2 mm beyond the margins of the lesion.
- For thicker lesions such as warts and hypertrophic actinic keratoses, the application time is 10 to 30 seconds.

Spray Technique

- Spray the lesion until a full ice ball can be seen. The spray can be controlled with different-sized nozzles supplied with the equipment.

Figure 79–1 Pressurized liquid nitrogen spray canister.

Tissue damage can be further controlled by spraying through otoscope speculums or neoprene cones placed around the lesion on the skin. This allows vigorous treatment and deeper damage to the lesion while limiting lateral destruction to surrounding skin.

- For thin lesions, 3 to 5 seconds of continuous spray is adequate.
- For thicker lesions, freeze for 5 to 20 seconds. For deep warts, as much as a 60- to 90-second freeze time may be required. A 1- to 3-mm halo of freeze around lesions usually ensures an adequate depth of injury.
- A word of advice: using many short bursts instead of a few prolonged sprays achieves only minimal tissue penetration. This is inadequate for treating thick lesions. However, it is wise for beginners to err on the side of undertreatment. A partially removed lesion can be retreated, but a scar cannot be eliminated.

WOUND CARE INSTRUCTIONS TO PATIENTS

It is most important to tell patients to expect that superficial lesions will be inflamed for 3 to 7 days and that thicker lesions often blister and contain clear or bloody fluid after treatment. Patients may be taught to sterilize a needle and drain the blister. The roof of the blister should be kept on to serve as an excellent biologic dressing while second-intention healing is under way. Thick lesions take approximately 2 weeks to heal.

Chapter 80

ELECTRODESICCATION AND CURETTAGE

David J. Leffell

Equipment needed
- Antiseptic solution
- 1% lidocaine with/without epinephrine 1:100,000 solution
- Curette (sizes 3 mm to 5 mm)
- Electrosurgical unit
- Sterile bandage
- Bacitracin/polymyxin ointment

CONSIDERATIONS

Electrodesiccation and curettage (EDC) is a useful technique for treating benign, superficial lesions, such as seborrheic keratoses or molluscum contagiosum. EDC can also be used to treat small and superficial basal cell or squamous cell carcinomas. Electrodesiccation refers to directing electric current to the skin surface with a monopolar electrode resulting in the destruction of the area. Cell death and tissue necrosis extend beyond the clinically detectable tumor margins, a process that effectively destroys residual malignant cells. EDC is not as effective as excisional surgery for curing basal cell or squamous cell carcinomas. However, the ease of the procedure, together with the lower cost and less invasive nature, may justify its use when treating small superficial tumors with clearly visible margins.

PROCEDURE

- Prepare the lesion and surrounding skin with antiseptic solution.
- Anesthetize the site with lidocaine 1% with or without epinephrine (1:100,000). Do not use epinephrine on the digits or on the tip of the penis. It is safe, however, on the nasal tip and ears. Epinephrine can reduce bleeding and make visualization of the lesion easier. The anesthetic effect may be almost immediate, but it is best to wait 3 to 5 minutes before proceeding. The full hemostatic effect takes somewhat longer to occur and helps to maintain hemostasis after the procedure.
- Make sure to anesthetize beyond the visible margins of the lesion because successive cycles of EDC will produce a wider area of tissue damage and charring.
- Start the EDC cycles by initially electrofulgurating the surface. That is, hold the electrode a fraction of a millimeter off the surface of the skin. This effectively removes the epidermal component, which can then be wiped clean with a gauze pad. Residual cancer is often detectable.
- Curette the tumor gently and extend curettage beyond the obvious area approximately 3 to 5 mm. Note the difference in the feel of the tumor compared with the noninvolved surrounding skin. Basal cell carcinomas tend to feel soft or gelatinous. One can often distinguish the margins of the tumor by feel alone.
- Electrodesiccate the entire base of the curetted area.

- Gently curette the surface again to remove the char, and repeat this cycle up to three times depending on the depth of the tumor.
- The wound bed should be curetted clean with no visible char, active bleeding, or oozing.
- Dress the area with topical antibiotic ointment, and cover the wound with a nonadherent dressing.

WOUND CARE INSTRUCTIONS TO PATIENT

Clean the wound daily with soap and tap water. Apply topical antibiotic ointment and cover the wound under a nonadherent dressing. This should be done until the wound is healed completely. Depending on the location, depth of treatment and quality of wound care, this can be from 5 days (locations above the neck) to 14 days (extremities). The healed EDC site may produce a round, hypopigmented, and slightly depressed scar. The scar becomes smaller in time but can be a concern to patients when it is prominent.

The following colleagues contributed greatly to the photography in this book. Their photos are used by their permission and as a courtesy; they retain all copyright privileges to their photographs published in this book.

I add a special note of thanks to Drs. Robert J. Cohen (New York University) and Mark G. Lebwohl (Mount Sinai School of Medicine), who generously allowed me to review their vast and excellent collections.

Figures 5–2, 9–1, 32–1 courtesy of Hilary Baldwin.

Figures 4–1, 8–1, 10–1, 13–1, 13–2, 14–1, 14–2, 15–2, 26–1, 30–1, 30–2, 31–1, 31–2, 31–3, 38–1, 60–1, 61–1, 62–1, 63–1, 64–1, 64–2, 65–1, 65–2, 66–1, 67–1 courtesy of Jeffrey P. Callen.

Figures 4–2, 20–2, 21–1, 21–2, 23–2, 29–1, 34–1, 35–1, 36–3, 36–4, 37–1, 39–1, 41–1, 42–1, 43–1, 49–1, 50–1, 58–1, 69–1, 74–1, 74–2, 76–1 courtesy of Robert J. Cohen.

Figures 25–1, 25–2, 33–1, 51–1, 54–1, 55–1, 56–1, 59–1, 59–2, 59–3, 70–1 courtesy of John T. Crissey.

Figure 22–2, courtesy of Drore Eisen.

Figures 23–1, 23–3, 24–2 courtesy of Donald Greer.

Figures 40–1, 45–1, 47–1 courtesy of Hossein Nousari.

Figures 9–2, 18–2 courtesy of The Lancet.

Figures 1–1, 6–1, 12–1, 20–1, 27–1, 27–2, 44–1, 48–1, 57–1, 68–1, 70–2, 71–1, 72–1, 73-1, 75-1, courtesy of Mark G. Lebwohl.

Figures 16–2, 17–1, 22–1, 24–1 courtesy of Larry E. Millikan.

Figure 18–1 courtesy of Robert Nadelman.

Figure 15–1 courtesy of Nicholas Soter.

Figures 2–1, 2–2, 2–3, courtesy of Amy Paller.

Figures 3–1, 2–4, 4–3, 19–1 courtesy of Lawrence Charles Parish.

Figures 5–1, 8–2, 11–1, 16–1, 20–3, 28–3, 36–1, 36–2, 37–2, 39–2, 39–3, 46–1, 52–1, 68–2 courtesy of James C. Shaw.

Figures 7–1, 28–1, 28–2, 40–2, 53–1 courtesy of Leonard Swinyer.

Figure 79–1 courtesy of Brymill Cryogenic Systems.

David H. Frankel, M.D.

INDEX